FORMULARY of PERFUMES and COSMETICS

by

R. M. GATTEFOSSÉ

Translated from the French

1959

CHEMICAL PUBLISHING CO., INC.

212 Fifth Avenue, New York, N. Y.

FIRST AMERICAN EDITION
1959

Printed in the United States of America

CONTENTS

3. *Various Types of Perfumes*

FORMULARY OF COSMETOLOGY

1. *Beauty Creams*

2. *Cosmetic Specialties for Holidays*

3. *Rouges*

4. *Lotions*

5. *Dentifrices*

6. *Hair Products*

7. *Nail Preparations*

INTRODUCTION

THE first editions of our formulary, especially those of 1911 and 1920, had their merit; it was then a question of choosing and devising a new approach.

Synthetic perfumes and terpeneless oils first appeared on the market as curiosities, and flower absolutes extracted with volatile solvents had hardly begun to replace pomades or enfleurage oils.

These new products appeared both daring and somewhat startling to manufacturers who, still steeped in a mysterious, traditional technique, were using a great variety of incompatible ingredients.

We assumed, then, that they were a mark of progress and simplification; did they not show a common characteristic of maximum concentration? Unit weight of the synthetic perfume was practically equal in fragrancy strength to a similar unit of the flower extract obtained with volatile solvents or to unit weight of terpeneless oil from which the less active hydrocarbon components had been removed in dilute alcohol.

Because of these new maximum strength fragrant materials there was no need to standardise the pomade washings whose "number" only indicated the number of kilogrammes of flowers used in their preparation and not the actual concentration; it was also necessary to ascertain the odour strength of fragrant oils; the uniformity of strength of the main raw materials allowed the preparation of a 100 per cent. composition of odorous preparations even if made up from raw materials from a variety of sources.

Some expensive synthetic perfumes—*e.g.*, ionone—were still sold in alcoholic solution; some crystalline products—*e.g.*, synthetic musks—were blended with several times their weight of inert odourless materials. The manufacturers had to be stimulated into supplying only pure materials.

The perfume manufacturers and chemists soon realised where their interests lay and barely ten years were required to crystallise the views which gave the French perfume industry its superiority. Thus a new industry of completely artificial perfumes was born. These perfumes only required dilution with alcohol to yield commercial products such as extracts, lotions, etc. The factories found it a rich source of business, especially the export to countries in which the French "composition" still enjoyed very great favour.

The wars, however, had a terrible effect on our national industries; while we were busy defending our land and later regaining our liberty, foreign factories, more favourably situated than ours, exerted themselves to satisfy the world-wide demand of customers and to supplant us. To what extent have they succeeded? The answer lies in the future.

We yet have our reputation; the main French perfumes are still recognised as the best by men and women of taste throughout the world.

The present formulary does not teach the compounding art; it is intended to keep the classical fundamental ideas, which we stressed in our earlier publications, constantly in front of manufacturers. The manual contains only typical examples of tested formulations and methods of preparation. It does not contain recipes which, slavishly followed, will yield perfumes similar to those of our great compounders.

As perfumery is an art, it should be revealed to artists; oil, or water-colour, painting manuals teach the holding of the brush and the spreading of colours, but not the art of producing a masterpiece. Our book will indicate how to handle odorant raw materials. If the compounder has talent and has acquired the technique of the art, then he will become an artist. When he has prepared a formula on the lines indicated in one of the subsequent chapters, and when he has memorised and classified the odours of various ingredients, he will be able to assess the smell of a composition and to relate it to his ideal; he will vary the proportions of the ingredients if he thinks it desirable, or he may replace some with other ingredients having a more subtle aroma. Ultimately he obtains the odour he desires, and if this odour pleases a large public he will become a "perfumer."

The manufacturer must realise that raw materials from different sources differ in their characteristics; essential oils are all vegetable products; there are essential oil soils just as there are vineyard soils. A common oil, like thyme, has its aroma affected by such factors as its botanical origin, its place and time of harvesting and its distillation. When this well-known flower is not well distilled an inferior oil results; if the distilled oil is unsuitably preserved, or if it is adulterated, deterioration will occur. Similar reservations apply to synthetic products; even though they are chemically pure they may lack faultless purity of odour; during their manufacture some fault, regarded as unimportant, may have arisen, but this fault nevertheless detracts from the perfume's final perfection. Lastly, the discovery of such odourless or practically odourless derivatives such as ethyl benzoate or benzyl benzoate permitted their use in blending, but by such blending the olfactory strengths of the ingredients are proportionately lowered. Watch must be kept on the quality and purity of the raw materials. A low price for an ingredient is not a criterion of its suitability; to the taster of fine wines and liqueurs price is a secondary consideration if their quality satisfies him.

The best perfumery formulations are not derived from the best formulæ; they are the inevitable result of the blending of faultless ingredients. One day it will be desirable to lay down specifications and limits for the origin of aromatic oils and to define their botanical classifications. After all, such specifications exist for branded chemical products.

A manual cannot impart this knowledge. It does, however, constantly remind us that perfumes cannot be made with ordinary ingredients of poor quality.

FORMULARY OF PERFUMERY

THE PERFUME INDUSTRY

WORKS like that of Felix Cola (*The Book of the Perfumer*) have taken a great place in the history of perfumery through the ages and civilisation. We recommend this book to readers who are anxious to further their knowledge of the connection between perfumery and culture. We are only concerned with practical laboratory hints. We shall consider also the philosophy of perfumes.

Perfumery products may be divided into three main classes:

Dilute alcoholic solutions.
Concentrated alcoholic solutions.
Alcohol-free products.

The first group comprises the lotions or toilet waters, the Colognes and lavender waters, incorrectly termed waters because they are alcoholic solutions.

Standard dilute alcohol 50-80° G.L. is generally used in their preparation. They may contain 1-2 per cent. perfume, sometimes more, sometimes less, according to the product's selling price and the concentration of the alcohol used in their preparation.

The second class comprises the extracts. They are prepared with 90° G.L. alcohol, so as to have a perfume content between 50 and 200 grammes per litre with a tendency to a still higher concentration. Maturing costs outstrip perfume prices.

The remaining class takes in alcohol-free, or almost alcohol-free, compositions intended for use in cosmetics and in the soap industry.

There have, of course, been considerable fundamental differences between various perfume compositions, particularly as regards their origin. So-called Cologne waters had a therapeutic purpose, like most aromatic waters created in the sixteenth and seventeenth centuries; the properties, flavour and odour determined the choice of essential oils for this purpose: this was so with the "Water of the Hungarian Queen," based on rosemary, as well as with "Angel Water" and many others.

Extracts mainly relied on their fragrance to please. The choice of ingredients only considered their purity and not their therapeutic properties.

They were also required to have very great persistency so that they would last the gala evening and night irrespective of whether dancing was indulged in or not.

These characteristics have to-day lost their importance. Skilfully formulated perfumes are used alike for extracts, toilet waters and lotions. The latter are included in the generic term "Flower Eaux-de-Cologne" or "Flowers of Fantasy." Diluted solutions should be described as "toilet waters" or "lotions," as otherwise the term Eau-de-Cologne loses its essential meaning. Terms such as these can only be altered slowly.

There is a tendency to use the same ingredients for luxury soaps as for perfumes of the alcoholic type. If such is the case alkali-stable ingredients must be introduced into the formulæ. At the same time the ingredients must be unaffected by the soaps themselves.

In brief, the technique is over-simplified and commercialised; the perfumer produces pure compounds and then he dissolves them in appropriate concentrations in more or less dilute alcohol, or other solvents!

It is useful to know how to substitute a highly priced ingredient by a cheaply priced one, without altering the odour of a particular composition; it is likewise useful to know how to choose an ingredient which is stable to soapy and non-soapy vehicles alike, and how to impart lasting qualities to perfumes—their fixation.

When reduced to such broad cut lines perfumery appears to be a simple art. In point of fact the manufacturer has to show more competence and attention to his work than ever he did, for the constantly increasing multiplicity of raw materials in regard to their botanical and geographical origins demands them.

Two substances may have a similar and possibly identical name. Let one instead of the other be used and there is trouble. There are still standard products—so called—which are sold every year. These products vary little from year to year.

The wines of Bercy, with their lack of individuality and aroma, were such "standard" materials.

There is full freedom to choose the "gros rouge" of Bourgogne or of Châteauneuf du Pape. But each, even the least expert, has his own likings. The faithful clientele of some commercial establishments in Paris like the selection in their cellars.

This applies to the perfumer with equal force. The user of

standard products has his customer, whereas he who has selected his materials with infinite care has a faithful, grateful clientele. Each will assume the position which appears the best. On the one hand will be chosen a dependable supplier for a particular but not outstanding product; on the other, suppliers of outstanding products, even when continuity of supplies are not assured, will be chosen because their products are so individualistic.

THE RAW MATERIALS OF THE PERFUMER

Some fifty years ago the perfumer's raw materials might have been classified into four groups:

1. Essential oils distilled from odoriferous plants, and aromatic waters, the residues from such distillation.
2. Alcoholic extracts of oils or fragrant pomades.
3. Resins and balsams.
4. Animal perfumes: musk, civet, castoreum and amber.

There are modern perfumery books that still use products embraced in the second category. We have simplified the classification by eliminating this class. They can, of course, still be used if due allowance is made for their "absolute perfume" content—*i.e.*, the aromatic constituents left after the solvent has been removed. They can then be regarded as standardised alcoholic tinctures of the absolute oils corresponding to enfleurage oils.

We now have a more extensive classification because new products and old are used side by side. The classification is:

1. Distilled essential oils, aromatic waters and their derivatives:
   (*a*) Terpeneless oils.
   (*b*) Pure natural constituents.
   (*c*) Perfumed waters.
2. Synthetic perfumes subdivided into derivatives of:
   (*a*) Coal.
   (*b*) Natural constituents.
3. Absolute flower-oils:
   (*a*) Absolutes in volatile solvents.
   (*b*) Enfleurage absolutes.
4. Resins, balsams and their derivatives. Their makers name them, *e.g.*, Resinaromas, Balsamaromas, Balsamodours, etc.

5. Animal Perfumes, musk, civet, amber, castoreum and their absolutes, freed from both insoluble and odourless materials.

We proceed at once to the consideration of formulæ for 100 per cent. synthetic compositions, for perfumers and manufacturers are well acquainted with these different materials.

PART I

SYNTHETIC PERFUMES AND 100 PER CENT. COMPOSITIONS

The perfumer now has at his command materials which are broadly comparable to one another, at least to a large extent, and which lend themselves to blending. He can prepare compositions, so called 100 per cent., which are free of alcohol or other solvent.

The final product consists solely of constituents, or materials from various sources, at maximum concentration. Chemists, engaged on syntheses, have anticipated such a possibility, and if the earlier chemists were content to prepare mixtures of chemically pure substances (synthetic and ingredients) and to anticipate consumers' wishes, succeeding chemists extended it. Natural essential oils (preferably terpeneless so as to avoid changing their solubility or their character), flower absolutes to improve their subtlety, and purified resins to impart permanence were added.

They have striven mainly to reconstruct the very expensive or rare flower essences, and they have used chemical analysis and analogy. They have vied with one another to prepare a synthetic jasmine comparable to the real absolute essence at a price equal to or more favourable than the price of the product in current use.

They made use of substances such as the acetate and other esters of benzyl alcohol, methyl anthranilate, ionone, cinnamic alcohol, etc.; they looked for new ingredients and made products from them. Some started an investigation of the jasmone ketone found in the natural oil; others replaced it by suitable amounts of fractions of ylang-ylang, rosewood, or geranium.

They prepared indol and then α-amyl-cinnamic aldehyde with the characteristic fatty odour of jasmine oil. Hydroxycitronellal used in the preparation of lilac, heliotropin with its flower odour, and eugenol derivatives were employed in such a composition. Lastly, the natural absolutes were introduced so that now a wide range of artificial jasmines is available to meet the most varied demands.

The chemist had prided himself in marketing his new synthetics; then, becoming aware of the importance his high quality synthetics had assumed, he kept some discoveries secret; these new secret compounds gave a highly original note to the compositions containing them. This eliminated any further competition until the time when the chemist of the rival firm discovered in his turn a new superior synthetic.

And so an intense rivalry ran through the synthetic manufacturers' factories. This was often a great advantage, particularly to well-organised firms who had the facilities for carrying out research work, but not to the perfumer, as had been the case formerly.

Thus the latter must buy his artificial perfume compounds from manufacturers. This is an asset to him, for as the proverb says, "In wishing to do everything one does nothing well."

The maker's primary prerogative of himself preparing his basic mixtures has passed from him to the perfumer who makes synthetics. But this surely ultimately benefits the quality. And again, the compounder need no longer cherish a museum of ingredients which might comprise an inactive stock, even though of great value.

The imitation of flower perfumes succeeded that of the natural flower essences. The natural essence of lilac, like others, had only been extracted out of curiosity. There followed a very large range of artificial essences: narcissus, sweet-pea, fern, heliotrope, cyclamen, honeysuckle, hawthorn, acacia, etc. The artificial flower essences, as well as the natural essences, facilitated the compounding of aromatic complexes which are the glory of our industry.

And then came "Bases," materials which cannot be used alone. Their odour cannot be likened to that of a flower. They impart an original but excellent note to mixtures of artificial and natural perfumes. These materials were given high-sounding names such as opoponax or panaxol, foam base with mushroom odour, wood, tobacco or leather "base."

These bases were mainly foundations to which lighter floral products were added to yield a very large variety of extremely pleasant aromas.

The exquisite novelties created in the interval between the two wars owed their origin to this development.

We reach the last stage in this gradual transformation through which the chemist became a perfumer, creating the many fragments of complexes which had only to be added in suitable amounts to alcohol. Occasionally it was necessary to add other ingredients to give the compositions a personal note.

The privileged composer's rôle reverts to the maker of synthetics. At his disposal are an infinite number of products as well as many secret substances. The chemist is surrounded by vast supplies of which no perfumer ever dreamt.

This is a pronounced disadvantage not only to our industry, but to the French perfumery art. The chemical factories supply both foreign and French firms, and if the latter do not maintain their artistic originality they run a risk of being gradually ousted from the position their predecessors gained against fierce rivalry.

The most anxious and representative of the profession, the independent manufacturers, the true creators and composers, know this well.

There is every reason to help and encourage new talent, but the practice of an art is something difficult, and outstanding personalities do not form the majority of those who patiently follow the trail. We shall reopen this question when opportunity offers.

Solubility Table of Terpeneless Essential Oils

1,000 *g. alcohol solvent approx. in grammes*

60°	70°	80°	*Terpeneless oil of*
50	100	1,500	Anet
5	25	850	Angelica
5	30	90	Anise
130	300	1,000	Great lavender
5	35	100	Chinese anise
10	30	200	Sweet Basil
150	500	2,500	Bay
60	300	1,200	Bergamot (orange)
100	300	1,250	Bitter orange
150	600	1,000	Rosewood
80	200	600	Cananga
100	500	1,800	Cinnamon (Ceylon)
200	1,100	3,000	Cinnamon leaves
80	450	1,300	Cardamom
150	300	1,900	Caraway
60	500	2,500	Cinnamon (Chinese)
2	5	15	Celery
3	20	1,450	Citronella grass
5	35	1,300	Lemon
200	300	1,200	Coriander
50	300	1,200	Cumin
7	15	200	Tarragon
10	50	150	Fennel
100	300	1,300	Geranium
300	800	1,300	Clove
100	350	1,800	Lavender
90	200	1,000	Lemongrass
10	300	600	Sweet lime
100	350	1,000	Laurel
2	15	1,300	Tangerine
10	25	1,100	Curled mint
80	300	950	Peppermint Mitcham
15	300	1,000	Peppermint French
18	300	900	American mint
60	300	1,000	Japanese mint
100	250	900	Myrtle
120	300	1,000	Bitter orange flowers
2	300	1,200	Sweet orange
100	300	600	Marjoram
60	300	1,200	Petitgrain
250	300	3,000	Pimento
2	—	12	Pine
2	15	20	Scotch pine
2	—	15	Pimelo pine
150	350	1,500	Rosemary
5	200	600	Sandalwood
10	40	150	Sassafras
10	450	1,000	Thyme
6	100	500	Vetiver
8	40	450	Ylang-ylang

Solubility Table of Principal Synthetic Perfumes

Designation	*Alcohol* 95°	70°	50°	*Vegetable oil*	*Mineral oil*	*Glycerine*	*Petroleum Jelly*	*Dist. Water*
Amyl acetate ..	500	—	—	300	50	—	50	—
Bornyl ,, ..	500	170	—	300	200	—	300	—
Citronelyl ,, ..	500	200	8	—	—	—	—	—
Geranyl ,, ..	500	140	1	300	200	—	300	—
Benzyl ,, ..	500	—	—	35	5	—	50	0·5
Linalyl ,, ..	500	70	2	300	200	—	300	—
Menthyl ,, ..	500	120	—	300	200	—	300	—
Terpenyl ,, ..	500	150	—	300	200	—	300	—
Benzoic acid ..	200	—	—	35	5	80	5	1·8
Cinnamic acid ..	20	—	—	10	—	—	—	0·4
Cinnamic alcohol	500	—	—	23	—	4	13	—
Phenylethyl ,,	500	—	—	200	60	10	5	15
Benzyl ,,	500	—	—	300	—	—	—	—
Anisaldehyde ..	500	450	80	70	8	—	30	—
Cinnamic aldehyde ..	500	20	—	300	15	—	80	—
Anethol	500	40	5	25	40	—	400	—
Borneol ..	500	80	6	300	—	—	300	—
Benzaldehyde ..	500	—	—	500	25	3	100	—
Methyl anthranilate ..	500	—	—	500	40	4	—	—
Benzyl benzoate ..	500	—	—	500	200	0·5	100	—
Citral	500	250	5	300	10	2	10	0·8
Coumarin ..	15	—	—	20	1	2	10	2
Eugenol	500	—	—	40	5	5	40	1
Geraniol ..	500	400	30	250	50	3	40	—
Heliotropine ..	160	120	60	180	10	15	15	1
Ionone	400	150	2	40	10	2	—	1
Hyacinth ..	500	—	—	—	40	10	30	1·5
Jasmine	500	—	—	500	40	8	150	1
Linalool	500	250	50	200	200	2	50	0·5
Lilac and Lily of the valley ..	500	200	50	200	50	3	40	1
Musk xylene ..	5	—	—	0·8	—	0·1		
Musk seed ..	25	—	—	—	—	—	—	—
Myrtol	30	10	—	10	10	0·5	10	0·5
Nerolin	200	—	—	25	35	2	3	—
Artificial orange flower ..	500	—	—	350	50	3	5	0·5
Artificial carnation ..	500	—	—	300	50	3	5	0·5
Rhodinol ..	500	200	—	300	30	5	4	1·5
Safrol	500	30	—	300	50	—	—	—
Terpineol ..	1,000	500	—	18	200	10	80	—
Yara-yara ..	20	—	—	20	12	5	5	0·1
Vanillin	200	200	—	20	7	—	7	0·8

The solubility in alcohol is correlated with the chemical function: alcohol 90° readily dissolves phenols and alcohols, and alcohol of lower strength dissolves them proportionally. The aromatic hydrocarbons are soluble only in strong alcohol; they are insoluble in alcohol of dilute strength. It will be found that in the case of esters derived from different alcohols but with the same acid radicle, the solubility decreases as the molecular weight increases. Where products contain both alcohols and esters, the least soluble are those with the greatest content of esters. The solubility in hydrocarbons—*e.g.*, petroleum oil—is generally the opposite to that in alcohol.

Table of Compositions of Most Frequently Used Essential Oils

Essence	*Usual concentration after deterpenation*	*Main ingredients*	*Percentage*		
			Terpene	*Resin*	*Odorant substances*
Bitter almond	1·5	Benzoic aldehyde	10-15	5-10	75-78
Anise	2	Anethol	10-15	5-10	75-90
Great lavender	2	Linalol, cineol	25-35	6-10	60
Azalea rosewood	2	Linalol	15-20	10	65
Chinese anise	2	Anethol	10-15	8	75-85
Bay	4	Chavicol	45-60	15-20	25-30
Bergamot (orange)	2·5	Linalyl acetate	55-60	10-35	35-45
Bitter orange	40	Citral	90-95	5	3-7
Birchwood	5		5-15	25	70
Cananga	3	Cadinene	25-60	15-20	25-55
Chinese cinnamon	2	Cinnamic aldehyde	15-20	20-30	50-60
Caraway	3	Carvone	30-60	2	35-60
Lemon	30	Citral	90-92	5-7	4-5
Citronella grass, Java	2	Geraniol, Citronellol	25-30	12-15	60-85
Cypress	20	Thujone, Alcohols	85-90	8	5-7
Tarragon	2	Estragol	25-35	2-5	60-70
Eucalyptus	2	Cineol	20-35	10	55-70
Sweet fennel	2	Fenone, Anethol	38-40	10	50
Geranium	2	Rhodinol	25-30	13-15	50
Clove	2	Eugenol	15-20	5-10	75-92
Lavender	2	Linalyl acetate	10-15	5	70
Lemongrass	2	Citral	25-30	18-20	55-78
Sweet lime	16	Citral	75-85	12-18	7-10
Linalool	2	Linalool	15-25	20-25	60-90
Myrtle	2	Myrtol	60-65	5-10	30
Mace	10	Alcohols and phenols	60-90	10	8-10
Marjoram	2	Terpineol and camphor	40-50	12	40
Mint, American	2	Menthol	25-35	2	60
Mint, English	2	Menthol	20-30	2-5	70
Mint, French	2	Menthol	20-30	2-5	70
Mint, Pennyroyal	1·5	Pulegone	10-25	2-5	80-90
Sweet orange	40	Citral, C_{10} Aldehyde	90-95	5	2-3
Marjoram	2·5	Thymol	50-65	8	40
Petitgrain	2	Linalool, Nerol	36-45	5-10	50
Rosemary	4	Borneol, Cineol	60-65	5-10	25
Rose	2	Geraniol, Citronellal	30-50	1-2	50-60
Sandalwood	2-3	Santalol	5-25	12	40-90
Sassafras	2	Safrol	10-20	2-5	75-80
Clary sage	2	Linalyl acetate	15-25	22	60
Thyme	2-5	Thymol, Carvacrol	50-60	7	25-45
Verbena	2·5	Citral	25-40	5-12	35-45
Vetiver	2·5	Vetiverol	1-5	20-40	30-60
Ylang-ylang	3-5	Methyl para cresol	1-5	30-60	15-60

Table of Constituents of Commercially Used Essential Oils

Name of constituent	*Chemical nature*	*Extract of*	*Use*
Benzoic acid	Acid	Benzoin. Synthesis from cresol	Fixer
Anisic alcohol	Alcohol	Chinese anise	Lilac odour
Cinnamic alcohol	Alcohol	Storax	Hyacinth odour
Nonylic acid	Acid	Sweet orange	Orange odour
Anisic aldehyde	Aldehyde	Chinese anise. Synthesis from cresol	Hawthorn odour
Benzaldehyde	Aldehyde	Bitter almond	Bitter almond
Cinnamic aldehyde	Aldehyde	Essence of Chinese cinnamon. Synthesis from benzaldehyde	Replacement of Chinese cinnamon
Anethol	Phenol	Essence of anise, Russian, Spanish, French, Chinese. Essence of fennel	Replacement of essence of anise
Aurantine Citrene Carvene Limonene	Terpenes	$C_{10}H_{16}$ terpenes with only a slight odour of their own	Solvents for soap perfumes
Borneol	Alcohol	Rosemary. Synthesis from turpentine	Pine odour. Fixer
Camphene	Terpene	Essence of camphor	Resinous odour of camphor
Camphor	Ketone	Camphor tree	Pharmaceutical camphor
Carvacrol	Phenol	Essence of thyme	Isomer of thymol
Caryophyllin	Oxide	Essence of clove	Terpene, pungent odour
Chavicol	Phenol	Bay	Bay odour
Cineol or eucalyptol	Oxide	Essence of eucalyptus, great lavender	Antiseptic
Citral	Aldehyde	Lemongrass. Lemon	Fifteen times as strong as lemon essence
Citronellol	Alcohol	Essence of rose. Geranium. Synthesis by reduction of citronellal	Rose base
Coumarin	Alcohol	Tonka bean, sweet clover. Synthesis from salicyl aldehyde	Strong fixer. For most extracts; perfumes for soaps and face powders
Eugenol	Phenol	Clove, pimento	Clove odour
Irone	Ketone	Root	Is replaced by active ionone
Geraniol	Alcohol	Rose, geranium	Rose "case" for soaps
Linalool	Alcohol	Linaloa, rosewood. Licari. Bergamot	Base for most perfumes
Menthol	Alcohol	Mint essence. Synthesis	Replaces mint essence
Methyl heptenone	Ketone	Lemongrass essence	Very faint verbena odour
Nerol	Alcohol	Petitgrain, orange flower, rose	Odour of rose, orange
Pinene	Terpene	Turpentine, essence of wood	Turpentine and pine odour
Rhodinol	Alcohol	Geranium, rose	Fine odour of rose
Safrol	Phenol	Sassafras, essence of camphor	Wood odour. Raw material for heliotropin
Santalol	Alcohol	Sandalwood	Fixer. Sweet odour of wood
Styrol	Alcohol	Styrax	Fixer. Strong odour
Terpineol	Alcohol	Pine oil or synthesis	Lilac odour
Thujone	Ketone	Absinthe	Strong herbaceous odour
Thymene	Terpene	Thyme. Ajowan	Solvent
Thymol	Phenol	Thyme or Ajowan or synthesis	Antiseptic

Comparison between Solubilities of Essential Oils and Terpeneless Essences

Name of essence	*Solubility of the essential oil*		*Solubility of terpeneless essences*	
Bitter orange	Volumes 5-19	90°	Volumes 2	70°
Chinese anise	,, 10-15	90°	,, 6-10	80°
Chinese cinnamon	,, 20	70°	,, 6	60°
Cinnamon leaves	,, 5	70°	,, 3·5	60°
Cardamom	not soluble at 65°		,, 35	60°
Caraway	Volumes 15	75°	,, 2	70°
Celery	,, 10	90°	,, 2-4	70°
Lemon	,, 2	96°	,, 2	70°
Citronella, Ceylon	,, 1·3	80°	,, 0·5	80°
Citronella, Java	,, 4·5	80°	,, 0·8	80°
Cumin	,, 10	80°	,, 1	80°
Cypress	,, 18	80°	,, 1	80°
Juniper tree	,, 10	90°	,, 1·5	80°
Hyssop	,, 650	70°	,, 45	70°
Tangerine	,, 10	90°	,, 1	80°
Mint	,, 5	70°	,, 2-5	70°
Patchouli	,, 10	91°	,, 3	80°
Rosemary	,, 10	80°	,, 1	80°
Ylang-ylang	,, 2	90°	,, 1	80°

The figures indicate the millilitres of alcohol of the strength given that are required to dissolve 1 millilitre of perfume.

Table of Concentration of Terpeneless Essences (after H. Haensel)

	Times
French anise	2
Lavender	2
Chinese anise	2
Basil	2·5
Bay	4
Bergamot (orange)	2-3
Rosewood	2
Bitter orange	40
Rhodes bark	3
Calamus	8
Cananga	2-3
Cinnamon	2-3
Caraway	3
Lemon citron	30-40
Lemon	20-30
Citronella	2
Coriander	4
Cumin	4
Cypress	20
Eucalyptus	2
Fennel	2
Juniper bay	20
Geranium	2
Ginger	8
Gingergrass	2
Clove	2
Hyssop	2-4
Lavender	2
Laurel	4
Lemongrass	2
Lime (sweet)	20
Linaloa	2
Mace	4
Tangerine	70
Marjoram	2
Balm mint	5
Mint	2
Nutmeg	4
Myrtle	3
Orange flower	3
Orange sweet	40
Marjoram	2·5
Palmarosa	2
Patchouli	2
Petitgrain	2
Rosemary	4
Rue	2
Sandalwood	3
Pepperwort	3
Sage (common)	2
Sage (clary)	2
Thyme (wild)	4-10
Thyme	3-5
Tansy	2
Verbena	2·5
Vetiver	3-5
Ylang-ylang	2-6

Floral Compositions

We sought to group the various odours into families in order to facilitate their study and classification. While these groups are clearly anomalous botanically, they do consist of odours which are similar from the olfactory point of view, and they do permit consideration of their syntheses and their simulation with synthetic products.

A considerable number of groups can be formed, particularly if we take into consideration the odours which are of no direct interest to the manufacturer. Cerbelaud created 45 divisions, but it is possible to lessen this number by adopting an objective practical outlook. We ourselves have retained but 15 of them. Despite this there are many typical odours such as mint, anise, lavender, which do not lend themselves to imitation by means of synthetics. Moreover, they do not justify the work involved in their synthesis, particularly because of the shortage of the raw materials in present circumstances, and, additionally, the cost of the synthetic product would be greater than that of the natural product.

The manufacturer will readily distinguish between the recipes we quote. Some are essentially products made up from synthetics or from constituents of the natural oils, others are improvements. We draw attention to those made from synthetic complexes, to be diluted later with alcohol to form the final product, and to others which are "developed." In the latter are successively indicated the essential synthetics and the natural adjuvants or other ingredients which improve the products.

It is necessary to dilute such compositions to obtain their full value, and for this purpose "pre-fixed" alcohol is used. Such alcohol is prepared by adding to the solvent tinctures of amber or genuine musk or even fixers, but not mixtures of artificial musk, orange bergamot and ethyl phthalate.

A well-compounded perfume usually consists of three odours: that which is first perceived, a second floral portion harmoniously composed, and the third, the base or fixative. This base odour must be persistent, tenacious and accentuating without marring or masking the initial sensation.

We shall come back to this when artistic compositions are discussed. We did, however, deem it necessary to make this clear before the study of the following recipes was initiated.

Table of Floral Families

Notes	*Families*	*Natural complexes*
Benzyl acetate (and other benzyl esters) Hydroxycitronellol Terpineol Linalool Jasmine aldehyde	1. Jasmine-like Jasmine Lilac Lily of the valley	Essence of jasmine ,, ylang - ylang Artificial lilac, lily of the valley
Nerol Methyl anthranilate Farnesol	2. Orange	Essence of Neroli ,, orange flower ,, petitgrain ,, acacia
Paracresyl esters Phenylacetic esters	3. Narcissus Tuberose	Essence of tuberose ,, jonquil ,, broom
Phenylethyl alcohol Geraniol Citronellol Rhodinol Diphenyl oxide	4. Rose Geranium	Essence of solid distilled rose ,, geranium ,, palmarosa
Irone Ionone Methyl ionone Methyl heptine carbonate	5. Violet	Essence of violet ,, mignonette ,, iris
Paramethylacetophenone	6. Mimosa	Essence of cassia ,, mimosa
Citral Citronellal Citrene or Limonene	7. Lemon	Essence of lemon ,, verbena ,, palm mint
C_{10}-aldehyde Methyl anthrarilate	8. Aurantiæ	Essence of orange ,, tangerine ,, lemon
Terpenyl acetate Linalyl acetate Linalyl esters	9. Lavender	Essence of lavender ,, great lavender ,, hyssop ,, laurel
Pulegone Menthol Menthone	10. Mint	Essence of mint
Cinnamic aldehyde Eugenol Thymol	11. Spice	Essence of cinnamon ,, clove ,, bay ,, tarragon ,, thyme
Borneol and acetate Camphor	12. Woods	Essence of pine ,, juniper ,, rosemary
Vanillin Heliotropin	13. Vanilla	
Anethol	14. Anise	Essence of anise ,, fennel ,, Chinese anise
Clary sage Labdanum	15. Amber	Absolute of rock rose ,, oak moss

Family of Jasmines

Jasmine Variety

Jasmine is one of the most appreciated flowers because of its fine, sweet odour. Manufacturers seek to create imitations either by using commercial absolute essences or by carrying out research on the fresh flower itself.

Heine's classic patented (1902) formula is:

	Grammes
Jasmone	30
Linalyl acetate	150
Linalool	100
Benzyl acetate	550
Indole	25
Methyl anthranilate	5
Benzyl alcohol	140

The odourless benzyl alcohol which is now not used is readily replaceable by cinnamic alcohol with its sweet floral bouquet.

Jasmone, commercially unavailable, can be replaced in the formula with products having a jasmine-like odour or by ylang-ylang essence. A mixture of benzyl alcohol esters, such as the butyrate, acetate, propionate, etc., can also be used. Thus we obtain:

Artificial Jasmine I

	Grammes
Benzyl acetate	400
Benzyl butyrate	100
Essence of ylang-ylang	250
α-Ionone	50
Methyl anthranilate	25
Heliotropin	25
Cinnamic alcohol	150

Enfleurage products sometimes have a fatty odour and so *a*-cinnamic aldehyde, discovered by Descollenges and named Flosal, is used in their stead.

Artificial Jasmine II

	Grammes
Benzyl acetate	400
Benzyl propionate	10
Linalool and its acetate	180
Cinnamic alcohol	90
Cinnamyl acetate	20
Phenyl ethyl alcohol	50
Methyl anthranilate	20
Propyl acetate	30
Cinnamic amyl aldehyde	70
Ylang-ylang essence	100
Absolute jasmine essence	20

The manufacturer can vary the proportions to his taste. The rose-like characteristic can be accentuated and new constituents added.

Artificial Jasmine III

	Grammes
Benzyl acetate	300
Benzyl butyrate	15
Benzyl formate	15
Benzyl salicylate	30
Phenyl ethyl alcohol	50
Cinnamic alcohol	50
Cinnamic amyl aldehyde	35
Linalyl acetate	25
Hydroxycitronellal	65
Essence of ylang-ylang	200
Geraniol	60
Absolute jasmine, petroleum	35
Absolute jasmine, enfleurage	50

Sometimes stronger concentrations of hydroxycitronellal are used, and yet the lilac-like aroma of the product, although pleasant, is nevertheless different from that of jasmine.

The odour of lilac is obtained by this change.

Jasmine Complex IV

	Grammes
Artificial jasmine	465
Rhodinol	120
Heliotropin	90
α-Ionone	60
Ylang-ylang essence	100
Absolute jasmine essence	90
Musk ketone	50
Hydroxycitronellal	50

Jasmine (English) V
(according to W. A. Poucher)

	Grammes
Benzyl acetate	200
Linalool	100
Hydroxycitronellal	250
Phenyl ethyl alcohol	100
Phenyl ethyl iso-butyrate	90
α-Ionone	50
Cinnamic amyl aldehyde	30
Ylang-ylang portion	20
Phenyl acetic aldehyde	10
Benzyl salicylate	50
Indol	1
C_{10} aldehyde (10 per cent.)	3
Octyl iso-butyrate	1
Paracresyl phenyl acetate	30
Jasmone	10
Jasmine absolute	30
Civet	5
Musk ketone	20

Jasmine VI

	Grammes
Benzyl acetate	300
Benzyl formate	30
Linalyl acetate	150
Linalool	100
Methyl anthranilate	50
Hydroxycitronellal	100
Cinnamic amyl aldehyde	100
Ylang-ylang essence	30
Nerol	10
C_{10}-aldehyde (10 per cent.)	10
Jasmine base	70

Jasmine VII

	Grammes
Benzyl acetate	300
Cinnamic alcohol	50
Linalool	50
Linalyl acetate	110
Phenyl ethyl alcohol	30
Methyl ionone	100
Ylang-ylang essence	25
Synthetic peach	5
Amyl cinnamic aldehyde	30
Hydroxycitronellal	200
Jasmine aldehyde	100

Jasmine VIII

	Grammes
Benzyl acetate	360
Linalyl acetate	60
Phenyl ethyl alcohol	60
Amyl cinnamic alcohol	90
Hydroxycitronellal	100
Benzyl alcohol	80
Methyl anthranilate	30
Linalool	45
Paracresyl phenacetate	15
Cananga essence	50
Sandalwood essence	30
Dimethyl benzyl carbinol	15
Resinodor storax	50
Benzyl formate	15

Jasmine Super IX

	Grammes
Artificial jasmine	465
Jasmine absolute	20
Ylang-ylang essence (Bourbon)	100
Rhodinol (pure)	120
Heliotropin	90
α-Ionone	60
Linalool	45
Hydroxycitronellal	50
Musk ketone	50

Lily of the Valley III

	Grammes
Hydroxycitronellal	350
Dimethyl benzyl carbinol	180
Phenyl ethyl alcohol	60
Ionone	30
Terpineol	200
Citronellol	30
Cinnamic alcohol	50
Heliotropin	30
Ylang-ylang essence	50
Rosewood essence	50
Vanillin	5

Lily of the Valley (English) IV (after W. A. Poucher)

	Grammes
Terpineol	100
Linalol	150
Hydroxycitronellal	250
Amyl cinnamic aldehyde	50
Citronellol	100
Phenyl propyl alcohol	30
Phenyl ethyl salicylate	50
Artificial jasmine	90
Bergamot (orange) essence	100
Ylang-ylang essence	20
Neroli essence	10
Tuberose absolute	10

Lily of the Valley Super V

	Grammes
Artificial lily of the valley	700
Hydroxycitronellal	25
Rhodinol	60
Jasmine absolute	10
Jasmine (synthetic) extra	40
Linalol	25
Heliotropin	80
Vanillin	10
Musk xylene	50

Lily of the Valley Super VI

	Grammes
Lily of the valley (artificial)	600
Hydroxycitronellal	200
Linalol	20
Rhodinol	45
Jasmine absolute	5
Phenylethyl alcohol	50
Vanillin	35
Musk ambrette	45

Lily of the Valley VII

	Grammes
Lily of the valley (artificial)	680
Hydroxycitronellal	25
Rhodinol	60
Vanillin	10
Linalol	25
Heliotropin	80
Musk xylene	50
Jasmine absolute	10
C_9-C_{10}-aldehyde	10
C_9-aldehyde	10

Lily of the Valley VIII

	Grammes
Lily of the valley (artificial)	600
Hydroxycitronellal	200
Linalol	20
Rhodinol	45
Phenylethyl alcohol	50
Vanillin	50
Musk ambrette	25
Jasmine absolute	5

Cyclamen, despite its specifically crude aroma unless it is carefully prepared, can be used.

Cyclamen Variety

Cyclamen I

	Grammes
Hydroxycitronellal	250
Cinnamic alcohol	200
Benzyl acetate	50
Phenylacetic aldehyde	2
Rhodinol	80
Citronellol	150
Farnesol or dimethyl octanol	30
Amyl cinnamic aldehyde	25
Phenyl ethyl acetate	60
Heliotropin	100
C_{10}-aldehyde	3
Bulgarian rose (pure)	50

Cyclamen Super II

	Grammes
Cyclamen (artificial, *vide supra*)	455
Lilac (artificial, extra)	160
Bulgarian rose (essence)	20
Ylang-ylang essence	40
Jasmine (artificial)	45
Jasmine (absolute)	10
Hydroxycitronellal	75
α-Ionone	30
Citronellol	60
Coumarin	30
Musk ketone	50
C_{10}-aldehyde (pure)	5

Cyclamen III

	Grammes
Cyclamen (artificial)	460
Lilac (artificial)	160
Hydroxycitronellal	75
Jasmine (artificial)	45
Ylang-ylang	40
α-Ionone	30
Citronellol	60
Coumarin	30
Musk ketone	50
Bulgarian rose (essence)	20
Jasmine absolute	10

Mock Orange

	Grammes
Jasmine (artificial)	500
Lily of the valley (artificial)	365
Methylnaphthyl ketone (D)	25
Methyl ionone	50
Orange-flower petals essence	50
C_9-C_{10} aldehyde	10

Ylang-Ylang Variety

Ylang-ylang I

	Grammes
Ylang-ylang essence	600
Jasmine (artificial)	300
Bulgarian rose essence	40
Moroccan cedar essence	60

Ylang-ylang II

	Grammes
Ylang-ylang essence	640
Lilac (artificial)	200
Lily of the valley (artificial)	60
Hydroxycitronellal	90
Jasmine (artificial)	50
Heliotropin	60
Vanillin	10
Benzyl salicylate	60
Musk ambrette	20
Jasmine absolute	10

Ylang-ylang III for Extracts

	Grammes
Ylang-ylang essence, Bourbon extra	630
Lilac flower (artificial)	200
Lily of the valley flowers (artificial)	60
Hydroxycitronellal	90
Jasmine flowers essence	50
Jasmine absolute	10
Benzyl salicylate	60
Heliotropin	60
Vanillin	10
Clary sage	10
Musk ambrette	10
C_{10}-aldehyde	10

Bouvardia

	Grammes
Phenylethyl alcohol	100
Rosewood essence	100
Methyl ionone	325
Iso-eugenol	100
Cinnamic alcohol (storax)	225
Citronellol	75
α-Ionone	70
Methyl heptine carbonate	5

Amaryllis

	Grammes
Hydroxycitronellal	300
Terpineol	300
Ylang-ylang essence	50
Neroli essence	50
Artificial rose essence	30
Rosewood essence	200
Sandalwood essence	50
Vanillin	4
Hendecalactone	1
Musk ketone	15

Orange Family

The orange family embraces neroli, obtained from the blossoms by distillation, and oil of petitgrain, which is distilled from the young orange sprouts or leaves. Mandarin oils are characterised by their content of methyl anthranilate and of the methyl ester of methylanthranilic acid.

Synthetics having a similar odour are anthranilate, orange ketone, methyl naphthyl ketone and aurantiol, a condensation product of methyl anthranilate and hydroxycitronellal. Desirable orange bouquets, at various price levels, are prepared by adding the materials in suitable amounts to terpeneless petitgrain oil.

Neroli Variety

Artificial Neroli I

	Grammes
Petitgrain oil (terpeneless) bitter orange	600
Methyl anthranilate	18
Linalol	200
Farnesol	100
Methylnaphthyl ketone	20
Nonylic aldehyde	1
Decylic aldehyde	30
Aurantiol	30
Nerol	30

Artificial Neroli II

	Grammes
Petitgrain oil (terpeneless) ≡essence	300
Linalol (lavender)	200
Phenylethyl alcohol	100
Nerol	100
Lemon oil	80
Neroli oil (Portugal)	15
Hydroxycitronellal	50
Methyl anthranilate	50
Methyl ester of methyl anthranilic acid	50
Amyl cinnamic aldehyde	10
C_{10}-aldehyde	15
Methyl naphthyl ketone	60

Acacia and sweet pea are included by Cerbelaud in the orange family. A few examples follow:

Acacia Variety

Acacia I

	Grammes
Acaciol	700
Benzyl acetate	100
Phenylethyl alcohol	100
Amyl cinnamic aldehyde	83
Methyl salicylate	15
C_9-aldehyde	2

Acacia II

	Grammes
Acaciol	400
Linalol	200
Phenylethyl alcohol	100
Cinnamic alcohol	70
Ionone	80
Para-methylacetophenone	10
Methyl salicylate	15
Citronellol	60
Methyl naphthyl ketone	15
Bergamot oil (essence) orange	50

Acaciol is a condensation product of hydroxycitronellal and anisic aldehyde. If so desired the amount used can be reduced as the odour is distinctly insipid and slightly sickening.

Acacia III

	Grammes
Neroline	25
Rose absolute	10
Aurantiol	80
Phenyl ethyl alcohol	30
Linalol	20
Artificial jasmine (flower)	60
Bergamot oil (essence) orange	80
Artificial acacia	600
α-Ionone	65
C_9-C_{10}-aldehyde	10
Musk ketone	20

Acacia IV

	Grammes
Artificial acacia	570
Neroline	25
Aurantiol	80
Phenylethyl alcohol	30
Rosewood oil	20
Bergamot oil	80
α-Ionone	65
Jasmine flowers	60
Rose absolute	10
Musk ambrette	40
Musk ketone	20

Sweet Pea Variety

Essence of Sweet Pea had its period of popularity. It should be possible to obtain new effects with it. The English, who are more interested in it than we are, have achieved some very desirable variations.

It is essential to do without benzylidene acetone in sweet pea creations, for it is strongly irritant, particularly towards the mucous membranes of the nostrils.

Sweet Pea I

	Grammes
Dimethylbenzyl carbinol acetate	50
Phenylethyl acetate	50
Benzyl acetate	70
Cinnamic alcohol	200
Phenylethyl alcohol	200
Amyl cinnamic aldehyde	125
Phenylacetic aldehyde	3
Aurantiol	30
Essence of natural neroli	70
C_9, C_{10}, C_{12}-aldehydes	2

Sweet Pea II

	Grammes
Aurantiol	50
Hydroxycitronellal	120
Artificial sweet pea	620
Cinnamic alcohol	80
Neroli oil	20
Rose oil	60
Jasmine absolute	10
Musk ambrette	40

Sweet Pea III

	Grammes
Terpineol	265
Phenylacetic aldehyde	35
Bergamot oil	180
Guinea orange oil	50
Ylang-ylang	5
Linalol of lavandin	200
α-Ionone	50
Isobutyl phenylacetate	40
Orange flower absolute	50
Methyl nonyl acetic acid, 10 per cent.	5
Methyl naphthyl ketone	50
Heliotropin	68
Vanillin	2

Sweet Pea Super IV

	Grammes
Aurantiol	50
Hydroxycitronellal	120
Sweet pea (*vide supra*)	620
Jasmine absolute	10
Cinnamic alcohol	80
Neroli bitter orange	20
Rhodinol	60
Musk ambrette	40

Family of Narcissus

Since the paracresol esters were discovered it has been customary to prepare synthetic blends of the narcissus perfume. These pure products do not have particularly pleasant aromas, in fact their odours have been likened to that of buck-skin or to that of a stable. However, when they are blended with the ingredients used in the foregoing formulæ they give them quite original characteristics. Thus by blending together synthetic neroli, jasmine, lilac with paracresyl acetate or the meta- or para-cresyl derivative of phenyl acetic acid, a very good reproduction of a narcissus bouquet is obtained. Fancy perfumes can be obtained from this blend by mixing into it small amounts of such absolutes as Helichryse or Immortelle, Roman or Moroccan camomile, Clary Sage, Visnage, etc.

Bromostyrol and phenylacetic aldehyde form the basis of both jonquil and hyacinth odours. But they are gradually being ousted by cinnamic acid and its esters.

Narcissus Variety

Narcissus I

	Grammes
Synthetic neroli	700
Paracresyl acetate	5
Paracresyl phenylacetate	5
Methyl cinnamate	50
Cinnamic alcohol	200
Rose absolute	20
Jasmine absolute	20

Yellow Narcissus II

	Grammes
Artificial neroli	398
Citronellol	200
Ylang-ylang	100
Phenylethyl alcohol	200
Ethyl cinnamate	100
Metacresyl phenylacetate	2

Narcissus III

	Grammes
Terpineol	200
Linalol	100
Geraniol	100
Hydroxycitronellal	200
Paracresyl phenylacetate	80
Iso-eugenol	50
Petitgrain oil (terpeneless)	50
Phenylacetic aldehyde	20
Heliotropin	70
Benzyl acetate	130

Narcissus Super IV

	Grammes
Artificial narcissus as above	460
Sandalwood oil	60
Vetiver oil	40
Heliotropin	80
Vanillin	10
Artificial amber (pieces)	45
Neroli, bitter orange	80
Tuberose absolute	20
Jasmine absolute	10
Civet	10
Aqueous neroli extract	20
Jasmine absolute	20
Essence of costus	10
Artificial hyacinth	20
Methyl ionone	40
Benzyl salicylate	25
Phenylethyl alcohol	20
Aurantiol	10
Methyl, nonyl (or decyl) acetic aldehyde	10

Fancy Narcissus V

	Grammes
Essence of sandalwood	80
Neroli oil	20
Vetiver oil	125
Isobutyl salicylate	145
Phenylacetic aldehyde	50
Paracresyl acetate	200
Ylang-ylang	85
Heliotropin	55
Cinnamic alcohol	200

Hyacinth Variety

Hyacinth I

	Grammes
Artificial lilac	795
Essence of rosewood	200
Bromostyrol	2
Phenylacetic aldehyde	2
C_{11}-aldehyde	1

Hyacinth II

	Grammes
Artificial hyacinth	440
Cinnamic alcohol	60
Heliotropin	40
Hydroxycitronellal	75
Phenylethyl alcohol	65
Terpineol	95
Musk ketone	50
Essence of rose	50
Essence of jasmine absolute	75

Hyacinth III

	Grammes
Artificial lilac extra	400
Phenylacetic aldehyde	30
Rhodinol	100
Bulgarian rose	50
Jasmine absolute	35
Methyl ionone	120
Hydroxycitronellal	120
Heliotropin	40
Hyacinth absolute	60
Phenylethyl alcohol	20

Hyacinth Super IV

	Grammes
Artificial hyacinth as above	440
Cinnamic alcohol	60
Artificial rose	50
Artificial jasmine	75
Heliotropin	90
Hydroxycitronellal	75
Phenylethyl alcohol	65
Terpineol	95

Hyacinth V

	Grammes
Artificial lilac	500
Rhodinol	100
Methyl ionone	100
Hydroxycitronellal	115
Phenylacetic aldehyde	40
Bulgarian rose oil	50
Heliotropin	45
Phenylethyl alcohol	20
Hyacinth oil, absolute	20
C_8-C_{10}-aldehyde	10

Jonquil Variety

Jonquil I

	Grammes
Artificial neroli	500
Artificial lilac	470
Phenylethyl phenylacetate	25
Paracresyl phenylacetate	3
Methyl heptine carbonate	1
Phenylacetic aldehyde	1

Jonquil II

	Grammes
Terpineol	250
Linalol	250
Phenylethyl phenacetate	250
Phenylacetic aldehyde	50
Cinnamic alcohol	50
Iso-eugenol	50
Methyl cinnamate	20
C_{10}-aldehyde	10
Artificial jasmine extra	70

Clearly it is essential that we use the absolute essences (oils) in order to give quality to the preparations—*e.g.*, jonquil, hyacinth, orange-flower, jasmine and rose.

Glycine

Glycine has a sweeter odour; not only will the use of the paracresol esters be abandoned, but β-naphthyl ketone or orange ketone will be used in place of methyl anthranilate.

	Grammes
Neroli with ketone D	300
Artificial jasmine	300
Artificial cyclamen	200
Citronellol	50
Farnesol	50
Benzyl phenylacetate	30
C_8-C_{10}-aldehyde	10
Flower absolutes	60

Tuberoses belong to this family. The tuberose base which follows needs natural absolute essences of tuberose to round it off.

Tuberose

	Grammes
Ylang-ylang	200
Phenyl propyl alcohol	200
Methyl salicylate	10
Niobe oil	20
Benzyl acetate	50
Rosewood	60
Cinnamic alcohol	145
Methyl ionone	60
Methyl nonyl acetaldehyde 10 per cent.	10
Hydroxycitronellal	200
α-Ionone	45

Gardenia Variety

Gardenia I

	Grammes
Artificial lilac	400
Artificial jasmine	235
Citronellol	50
Acetyl iso-eugenol	35
Methyl heptine carbonate	5
Dimethyl benzyl carbinol	35
α-Ionone	100

Gardenia II

	Grammes
Artificial jasmine extra	420
Artificial lilac extra	165
Artificial rose	125
Artificial violet	80
Essence of bergamot	80
Iso-eugenol	40
Essence of sandalwood	15
Essence of styrolyl	15
C_{10}-aldehyde	2
C_{11}-aldehyde	2·5
Decyl alcohol acetate	0·5
Coumarin	15
Resinodour labdanum	15
Musk ketone	25

Gardenia III

	Grammes
Bergamot essence	120
Geranium essence	30
Ylang-ylang essence	30
Styrolyl acetate	80
Linalol	60
Cinnamic alcohol	60
Phenylethyl alcohol	120
Linalyl acetate	60
Cinnamyl acetate	60
Citronellyl acetate	60
Ionone	30
Hydroxycitronellal	80
Citronellol	60
Terpineol	90
Resinodour storax	60
Styrallyl acetate	90
Neroli	25
Rose absolute	25

Honeysuckle Variety

Honeysuckle I

	Grammes
Isobutyl phenylacetate	200
Cinnamic alcohol	185
Iso-eugenol	25
Synthetic jasmine	65
Ionone	160
Heliotropin	45
Vanillin	10
Artificial neroli	80
Rhodinol	60
C_{10}-C_{12}-aldehyde	10
Jasmine absolute	10
Orange flower absolute	10

Honeysuckle Super II

	Grammes
Synthetic honeysuckle as above	325
Orange flower absolute	10
Jasmine absolute	5
Artificial jasmine extra	65
α-Ionone	160
Heliotropin	45
Synthetic hyacinth	50
Vanillin	10
Petitgrain (Paraguay), terpeneless	20
Neroli, bitter orange	60
Synthetic civet	10
Rhodinol	60
Linalol	40
Cinnamic alcohol	95
Musk ketone	15
Musk ambrette	30

Magnolia

	Grammes
Ylang-ylang (composition)	350
Guaiacum	100
Citral	5
Linalyl acetate	50
Linalol lavandin	120
Anisic aldehyde	20
Methyl ionone	30
Hydroxycitronellal	45
Benzyl acetate	100
Amyl cinnamic aldehyde	75
Heliotropin	70
Musk ketone	30
C_{10}-aldehyde	5

Rose Family

There is an important place in perfumery for the many varieties of rose perfumes. The place may be more important than manufacturers think. In point of fact many formulæ contain quite large amounts of rhodinol, citronellol, geraniol, phenylethyl alcohol simply because of their aroma. These ingredients blend well with other substances—*e.g.*, ionones, methyl ionones, wood essences and jasmines—and yield very good reproductions.

When the formulæ of important fashionable perfumes are analysed it will be found that some of them contain synthetic rose essences to which the terms imperfect and extra classical can be applied. Again, as each flower has its own aroma, the rose lover, if he is a perfumer, can recall the years he spent in pursuit of the odours of his favourite flowers.

Rose perfume recipes of the formularies tend to give reproductions of classical odours—*e.g.*, distilled Bulgarian, French Rose, Red Rose or Brunner. The perfume is exquisite in the fresh flower: sometimes the odour is that of the White Rose—the Druschky, or that of the Yellow Rose—the Safrano.

Other rose compositions imitate with varying degrees of success such famous specialities as the Maréchal Niel Rose.

We may well ask ourselves whether rose recipes are still of interest, since floral extracts, despite their use in complex compositions, are not as highly regarded now as they were in the past.

Rose Base I

	Grammes
Rhodinol	285
Geraniol	145
Phenylethyl alcohol	430
Eugenol (from clove oil)	15
Bulgarian rose oil	125

Artificial Rose (Solid Type) II

	Grammes
Phenylethyl alcohol	400
Rhodinol	100
Tetrahydro-rhodinal	100
Citronellol	150
Concrete rose, absolute	250

Rose (Bulgarian Type) III

	Grammes
Geraniol from palmarosa	350
Geraniol from citronellol	250
Rhodinol	150
Phenylethyl alcohol	200
Essence (oil) of Bulgarian rose	50

Bulgarian Rose IV
(after W. A. Poucher)

	Grammes
Geraniol from palmarosa	400
Geranium oil (terpeneless)	60
Nerol	200
Phenylethyl alcohol	90
α-Ionone	40
Eugenol	10
Linalol	15
Geranyl acetate	35
Iris	10
Rhodinyl formate	20
Nonyl aldehyde C_9	1
Undecyl aldehyde C_{11}	2
Laurinic aldehyde C_{12}	2
Vanillin	7
Musk ketone	8
Bulgarian rose oil	100

Calyx Rose V

	Grammes
Essence (oil) of geranium (French, terpeneless)	530
Gingergrass oil (terpeneless)	35
Patchouli oil	45
Geraniol	55
Citronellol	20
Phenylethyl alcohol	75
Rhodinol	35
Linalol	65
Dimethylphenyl acetaldehyde	20
Phenylacetic aldehyde	50
Cinnamic aldehyde	70

Rose VI

	Grammes
Geranium oil (terpeneless)	180
Camomile oil (Moroccan, terpeneless)	60
Citronellol	360
Geranyl acetate	45
Nerol	15
Methyl ionone	15
Ionone	15
Phenylethyl alcohol	180
Isobutyl phenacetate	45
Rhodinol	60
Citronellyl acetate	40
Resinodour benzoin	30
Synthetic musk	15

Rose Super VII

	Grammes
Synthetic rose extra	500
Methyl ionone	100
Rhodinol	50
Phenylethyl alcohol	50
α-Ionone	60
Tincture of amber (20 per cent.)	60
Tincture of Tonkin musk (20 per cent.)	60
Jasmine absolute	20
Concrete iris (10 per cent. in alcohol)	20

Rose Super VIII

	Grammes
Artificial red rose	610
Moroccan rose absolute	40
α-Ionone	80
Methyl ionone	200
Jasmine absolute	10
Musk xylene	50
C_8-C_{10}-aldehyde	10

Red Rose IX

	Grammes
Rhodinol	250
Phenylethyl alcohol	100
Methyl ionone	100
Citronellyl formate	100
Bergamot	100
Synthetic jasmine	100
Cinnamic alcohol	80
Geranium (French, terpeneless)	65
Nonylic alcohol, C_9	4
Alcohol, C_{11}	1
Rhodinyl acetate	100

White Rose X

	Grammes
Palmarosa (terpeneless)	400
Gingergrass (terpeneless)	100
Geranium A (terpeneless)	50
Citronellol	150
Benzyl acetate	100
α-Ionone	60
Phenylethyl acetate	60
Phenylethyl alcohol	40
Nonylic alcohol	10
C_8-C_{10}-aldehyde	5
Patchouli (terpeneless)	5
δ-Methyl ionone	20

Rose for Extracts XI

	Grammes
Rose Brunner (100 per cent.)	500
δ-Methyl ionone	100
Rhodinol	50
Phenylethyl alcohol	50
α-Ionone	60
Iris tincture (10 per cent.)	20
Ambergris tincture (10 per cent.)	60
Tonkin musk tincture (10 per cent.)	60

Yellow Rose Safrano XII

	Grammes
Citronellol	350
Rhodinol	250
Phenylethyl alcohol	150
Farnesol or dimethyl octanol	10
α-Ionone	20
Guaiacol acetate	40
Crystalline cedrol	10
Heliotropin	50
Amyl cinnamic aldehyde	20

It is quite easy to vary these formulæ by making use of esters—*e.g.*, acetates and butyrates—of citronellol, rhodinol, geraniol, and farnesol. Nonylic aldehyde strengthens the odour, and makes it heavier.

Persian Rose XIV

	Grammes
Rose (100 per cent. synthetic)	920
Nerol	20
Nonylic aldehyde (10 per cent.)	15
Cedryl acetate	40
Citral	2
Phenylacetic aldehyde	3

Interesting new aromas can be developed by the use of such flower absolutes as jasmine mimosa, orange flower, etc. Very full vivid notes can be obtained by utilising geranium oils in the foregoing. The oils can be terpene-free, or not; the aroma of the oil is very much fuller and more vibrant than that of its individual constituents. The presence of geranyl tiglate in the natural oil undoubtedly contributes to this result.

It can be seen that the rose odours lend themselves to numerous permutations and so the reader is left to indulge himself in this pastime.

In a similar way the problem of geranium fragrances can be approached. The characteristic of a geranium composition is a leafy herbaceous odour, since geranium oils are mainly derived from leaves.

Natural geranium oils are used to give the geranium note, particularly as they are not costly. However, when they are to be used for the perfuming of ordinary soaps, natural oils or synthetic compositions, to which phenyl oxide or diphenyl methane is added, are used.

Violet Family

It has never been easy to prepare violet perfumes even when ionone was known. By the by, it is worth putting on record that the concentration of ionone affects its odour and that often the pleasant odour desired is lost because the optimum concentration is exceeded.

It is interesting to note that in 1907, when ionone was still sold as a 10 per cent. solution in alcohol at a high price, excellent preparations were frequently made. When, however, the price of ionone dropped, but its purity raised to 100 per cent., then the frequency of such good creations dropped. And the perfumers laid the blame on the chemists. They went so far as to increase the proportion of ionone; ionone has an odour of wood and shows a tendency towards acidity when used in large amounts.

Perfumers have tried methyl ionones as substitutes for iris, but they are difficult to use in effective proportions.

In order to obtain a very sweet composition for violet, use is very frequently made of such natural products as iris, ylang-ylang, cassia, mimosa, jasmine and violet leaves absolutes. The latter imparts the odour associated with violets when they begin to fade and are no longer giving off their natural scent. City inhabitants are more acquainted with this odour, whereas lovers of the countryside appreciate the more subtle one of freshly gathered flowers. Essences such as those of costus, umbelliferæ, carrots and visnage are sometimes used.

Every perfumer should thoroughly know and appreciate the odours of individual ionones, such as total ionone, α-ionone, β-ionone, the methyl ionones, di-hydro ionone, phenyl ionone, ianthone, alkyl cymyl ionone, as well as those of the specialities offered by inventors under fancy names. Nice leaf aromas are imparted by heptine and octine methyl carbonates.

Violet Variety

Violet Base I

	Grammes
α-Ionone	300
Methyl ionone	300
Ylang-ylang	50
Absolute of violet leaves	25
Absolute of cassia flowers	50
Resinoid of iris	50
Heliotropin	60
Bergamot	90
Jasmine absolute	30
Synthetic jasmine	25
Vetiver or Vetiverol	20

Wood Violet II

	Grammes
Violet base	400
α-Ionone	200
Synthetic jasmine flowers	200
Heliotropin	100
Bergamot	50
Musk xylene	50

Parma Violet III

	Grammes
Violet base	530
Methyl heptine carbonate	10
Synthetic jasmine	200
Cassia absolute	20
Liquid iris	100
Bergamot	60
Bulgarian rose	15
Vetiver composition oil	20
Civet absolute	5
Musk ketone	40

Common Violet IV

	Grammes
Total ionone	600
Anisic aldehyde	60
Synthetic jasmine	250
Synthetic rose	50
Octine methyl carbonate	5
Visnage	5
Musk ketone	30

Terpineol Violet V

	Grammes
Terpineol	380
Total ionone	300
Methyl ionone	100
Benzyl acetate	100
Methyl heptine carbonate	15
C_{12}-aldehyde	5
Heliotropin	100

Violet VI

	Grammes
α-Ionone	250
Methyl ionone	100
Bergamot	100
Ylang-ylang	40
Rose	5
Vetiver	40
Synthetic jasmine	200
Cassia absolute	25
Violet leaf absolute	4
Liquid iris	60
C_{12}-aldehyde	1
Heliotropin	75

Parma Violet VII

	Grammes
Total ionone	350
Methyl ionone	100
Synthetic jasmine	100
Hydroxycitronellal	40
Bergamot	100
Ylang-ylang	30
Liquid orris	100
Anisic aldehyde	40
Phenylethyl alcohol	60
Methyl heptine carbonate	10
Heliotropin	50
Concrete labdanum	17
C_{12}-aldehyde	3

Violet Super VIII

	Grammes
Synthetic violet extra	440
Absolute of violet leaves	20
Liquid orris	200
Cassia absolute	15
Bergamot	75
Bulgarian rose	15
Vetiver	20
Synthetic cassia	50
α-Ionone	120
Civet (pure)	5
Musk ketone	40

Violet IX

	Grammes
Total ionone	300
Methyl ionone	100
Liquid orris	100
Santalol	40
Methyl heptine carbonate	10
Absolute of violet leaves	20
Benzyl acetate	50
Citronellal	90
Ylang-ylang (terpeneless)	30
Bergamot	50
Phenylethyl alcohol	70
Vanillin	20
Benzyl alcohol	100
Musk ambrette	20

Liquid Violet X

	Grammes
α-Ionone	250
Methyl ionone	250
Ylang-ylang	50
Bergamot	90
Violet leaves	25
Jasmine absolute	30
Cassia absolute	50
Orris	50
Heliotropin	60
Synthetic jasmine	25
Tincture of civet (10 per cent.)	40
Tincture of musk tonquin (10 per cent.)	60
Vetiverol	20

Wood Violet XI

	Grammes
Synthetic violet extra	300
α-Ionone	250
Synthetic jasmine extra	150
Benzyl acetate	80
Heliotropin	130
Bergamot	90
Musk xylene	50

Iris (*Orris*)

	Grammes
α-Ionone	250
Methyl ionone	225
Resinoid of orris	75
Concrete orris	50
Vetiver	25
Crystalline cedrol	25
Anisic aldehyde	50
Terpineol	200
Heliotropin	50
Ethyl vanillin	10
Musk ketone	10

Mignonette Variety

Mignonette I (*Reseda*)

	Grammes
α-Ionone	250
Resinoid of orris	50
Methyl ionone	100
Phenylpropyl acetate	100
Geraniol (palmarosa)	200
Phenylethyl acetate	75
Styrallyl acetate	25
Methylnonyl ketone	25
Bergamot	75
Terpineol	100

Mignonette II (*Reseda*)

	Grammes
Methyl ionone	300
α-Ionone	50
Methyl heptine carbonate	10
C_{10}-C_{12}-aldehyde	20
Benzyl acetate	80
Bergamot	150
Petitgrain	80
Sweet Basil	10
Ylang-ylang (Bourbon)	30
Liquid orris	50
Mignonette (reseda) absolute	20
Linalol (lavandin)	100
Phenylpropyl alcohol	100

Mignonette III (*Reseda*)

	Grammes
Synthetic mignonette (reseda)	440
Phenylethyl acetate	80
Guaiacol acetate	90
Cinnamic alcohol	160
Synthetic carnation flowers	70
Santalol or cedrol	85
Methyl ionone	90
Vetiverol	40
Terpineol	60
Resinodour benzoin	75
C_{10}-C_{12}-aldehyde	5

Mimosa Family

Synthetic mimosas date from the discovery of paramethyl acetophenone, which is a characteristic ingredient of these preparations. There are numerous varieties, and by blending them it is possible to get some interesting results when used in combination with the foregoing recipes.

Cassia (*Acacia farnesiana*) has a fairly pure violet odour; the other species have a coumarin-like odour, sometimes with a bitter note.

Mimosa absolutes are of great value in many formulæ. Cuminic aldehyde imparts a pungent note. The methyl salicylate aroma of some species of mimosa is disliked by French customers.

Mimosa I

	Grammes
Terpineol	270
Cinnamic alcohol	200
Hydroxycitronellal	150
Anisic alcohol	70
Methyl acetophenone	120
Butyl salicylate	75
Linalol	70
Visnage	10
Heliotropin	30

Mimosa for Extracts II

	Grammes
Mimosa absolute	100
Artificial mimosa	125
Bulgarian rose	25
Ylang-ylang	70
Bergamot	60
Heliotropin	90
Coumarin	40
Isobutyl salicylate	95
Sandalwood	40
Synthetic civet	5
Musk ketone	50

Mimosa III

	Grammes
Paramethyl acetophenone	100
Terpineol	150
Hydroxycitronellal	100
Linalyl acetate	150
Ylang-ylang (Bourbon)	50
Cinnamic alcohol	100
Anisic aldehyde	20
Rhodinyl butyrate	25
Phenylacetic aldehyde	10
Amyl cinnamic aldehyde	60
Artificial rose	55
Artificial jasmine	80
Heliotropin	70
Musk ketone	30

Mimosa IV

	Grammes
Terpineol	200
Geraniol	150
Hydroxycitronellal	150
Acetophenone	80
Cuminic aldehyde	10
Benzyl acetate	100
Ylang-ylang	70
Methyl anthranilate	20
Phenylacetic aldehyde	10
Cinnamic alcohol	200

Mimosa Super V

	Grammes
Artificial mimosa as above	410
Natural mimosa absolute	100
Bulgarian rose	25
Ylang-ylang	70
Bergamot	60
Sandalwood	60
Heliotropin	90
Isobutyl salicylate	95
Synthetic civet	5
Coumarin	40
Musk ketone	50
C_9-C_{10}-aldehyde	10
C_{10}-C_{12}-aldehyde	5

Citrus Family

So many natural essences with the aroma of lemon, verbena or citronella (grass) are available that synthetics are wholly superfluous.

Lemongrass citral is frequently used as a base. Terpeneless lemon oil is a much better starting point, as not only is it free from terpenes but it is soluble in dilute alcohol. Either octyl or nonyl aldehydes can be used at low concentrations to reproduce the citral aroma.

Verbena

	Grammes
Verbena oil	150
Bergamot	140
Lemon	25
Rose	50
Artificial lilac flower	200
Rhodinol	125
Musk ketone	50
C_{10} aldehyde	10

Artificial Bergamot	*Grammes*
Bergamot	300
Terpenyl acetate	90
Linalyl acetate	112
Geranyl acetate	38
Linalol (lavandin)	75
Petitgrain oil (terpeneless)	120
Terpineol	190
Neroline	60
C_{10}-aldehyde	15

For Eaux-de-Cologne see special chapter dealing with them on pp. 57-63, 67-78.

AURANTIACEÆ FAMILY

The same comment applies to orange, tangerine and grapefruit aromas. Essence of bergamot is very often used to soften and round the crude odours of synthetics.

Bergamot can be replaced by synthetic linalyl acetate blended with orange (Guinea) and lemon oils and small quantities of neroli or petitgrain oil. This mixture of linalyl acetate together with other adjuvants gives a less insipid note than does rosewood acetate. The customer in general appears to have developed a partiality for lavender odours. We shall come back to this in the chapter on this family.

LAVENDER FAMILY

Natural essences with lavender odour are also quite numerous, so that a synthetic reproduction is really of no practical interest.

It is considered that the essential oils obtained from lavender grown at high altitudes are the best because of the high linalyl acetate content. This is not altogether true, for sometimes oils with a 35 per cent. content of this ester are better than those with 45 per cent. Again, each growth has an odour peculiar to itself. Thus essences from Diois have a very pleasant fruity odour; those from the Apt region are musty and their aroma is not unlike that of truffle; the essences from Vaucluse conform more to standard. The common varieties are quite neutral. Each perfumer can exercise his own choice of one or the other regional "crops."

The ordinary essential oils usually contain high proportions of the oil derived from Great Lavender—lavandin—a hybrid variety. The ester content of the oil is 20-30 per cent.; its odour, though crude, is sometimes preferable in well-balanced perfumes.

Great Lavender essential oils are resistant to deterioration, and because of this quality the oils are used in many important lavender perfumes. Rosemary oil also plays an interesting part, partly due to its floral aroma (in some ways rose-like, as its name suggests). But· again, the winter and spring essences differ from the summer essence in odour. Oils of common sage, hyssop and clary sage have an important role in the preparation of lavender perfumes; they are combined with lemon oils to give the freshness and key notes of all good perfumes.

Fern perfume has a complex yet lavender-like odour.

FERN VARIETY

Fern I

	Grammes
Lavender extra oil	200
Patchouli oil	15
Ylang-ylang	80
Rosemary	100
Rose compound	110
Bergamot oil	100
Jasmine compound	100
Oak-moss absolute	35
Lavender absolute in solvents	30
Heliotropin	100
Coumarin	70
Musk ketone	40
Methyl nonyl acetic, C_{10}-aldehyde	10

Fern II

	Grammes
Lavender oil	130
Patchouli oil	40
Ylang-ylang	100
Bergamot oil	110
Essence of oak moss	90
Rose absolute oil	25
Essence of concrete orris	25
Jasmine absolute oil	35
Rose artificial extra	135
α-Ionone	35
Coumarin	90
Heliotropin	125
Musk ketone	60

Readers are referred to the chapter on lavenders, waters and extracts, for further information.

MINT FAMILY

These essential oils are only used to a minor extent in perfumery. Small amounts are used in lotions to give them a particularly refreshing note.

Generally speaking, apart from the synthetic menthols, there are no synthetics with a mint-like odour.

Spice Family

Although the "spicy" note has not yet been evolved it must be emphasised that pungent odours can be just as important as those of wood and leather.

A very wide range of powerful, warm and clinging odours is offered by the essential oils of spices. These oils impart a slightly heavy oriental note to compositions in which they are incorporated, but their strength can be readily controlled by either using an appropriate amount, or by tact.

Hitherto eugenol, iso-eugenol and their esters have been used. Natural essences—*e.g.*, Amboine clove essence, Zanzibar clove oil, Madagascar clove oil—differ from one another in the subtlety of their aromas.

Highly original complexes result when these delicate tones are sought. Cinnamon oils vary widely, but it is not essential to use them at the expense of the clove oils. Cinnamic derivatives—*e.g.*, the cinnamic acid esters—belong to the same category despite their balsamic odour.

Zeodary, galanga, ginger, angelica, pepper, tarragon, safran, tonka, peppers, mace, nutmeg, juniper, cumin, coriander, celery, cardamom, calamus, caraway, bay, ambrette and others lend themselves to original, individual notes, and by making use of them, make commonplace compositions more outstanding.

Even with the extremely popular carnation family pleasant compositions can be made, and these can impart valuable variations to wood and leather tones.

Carnation Variety

White Carnation I

	Grammes
Isoeugenol	350
Benzyl isoeugenol	150
Rhodinol	90
Vanillin	25
Phenylethyl alcohol	130
Ylang-ylang	150
Bulgarian rose oil	75
Musk ketone	50

Red Carnation II

	Grammes
White carnation	510
Rhodinol	170
Eugenol	50
Methyl isoeugenol	40
Vanillin	40
Black pepper oil	35
Geranium oil (Bourbon)	90
Patchouli oil	15
Rose absolute	5
Musk ketone	50
Heliotropin	5

Carnation III

	Grammes
Isoeugenol	225
Acetyl isoeugenol	75
Eugenol	100
Phenylethyl alcohol	125
Cinnamic alcohol	225
Synthetic rose essence	100
Benzyl salicylate	100
Ionone	50

Carnation (English) IV (after W. A. Poucher)

	Grammes
Eugenol	300
Isoeugenol	200
Isobutyl phenylacetate	30
Benzyl isoeugenol	100
Hydroxycitronellal	20
Heliotropin	50
Terpineol	30
Phenylacetic aldehyde	10
Amyl salicylate	30
Phenylpropyl aldehyde	1
C_{10}-C_{16}-aldehyde	1
Vanillin	10
Petitgrain oil (terpeneless)	30
Rose oil	20
Ylang-ylang (terpeneless)	100
Nutmeg oil	18
Artificial jasmine	40

Carnation V (after W. A. Poucher)

	Grammes
Isoeugenol	250
Hexamethyl ketone	100
Heliotropin	20
Coumarin	20
Vanillin	20
Phenylpropyl aldehyde	1
Nerol	30
Amyl salicylate	60
Amboine clove oil	150
Clary sage oil	10
Pimento oil	100
Black pepper oil	19
Cananga oil	20
Cinnamon oil	10
Rose absolute essence	40
Resinodour benzoin	100
Musk ketone	20

White Carnation VI

	Grammes
Isoeugenol	250
Benzyl isoeugenol	150
Ylang-ylang (terpeneless)	150
Bulgarian rose oil	75
Clary sage oil	30
Synthetic cinnamic alcohol	120
Phenylethyl alcohol	60
Vanillin	25
Musk ketone	50
Rhodinol	70
C_9-C_{10}-aldehyde	20

Red Carnation VII

	Grammes
Synthetic carnation extra	420
Rhodinol	170
Rose absolute	5
Patchouli oil	15
Geranium oil (terpeneless)	90
Black pepper oil	25
Clary sage oil	45
Methyl isoeugenol	40
Vanillin	40
Heliotropin	5
Cinnamic alcohol	90
Musk ketone	55

Clover Aroma (English)

	Grammes
Bergamot oil	360
Vetiver oil	20
Ylang-ylang	160
Clove oil	40
Geranium oil	60
Coumarin	100
Vanillin	90
Amyl salicylate	100
Methyl acetophenone	20
Benzyl alcohol	50

Carnation VIII

	Grammes
Clove oil	400
Geranium oil	100
Cedar oil (soluble)	100
Bergamot oil	75
Isoeugenol	100
Amyl salicylate	55
Terpineol	120
Heliotropin	50

Oriental Perfume	*Grammes*
Oil of myrrh	80
Cardamom oil	20
Patchouli oil	40
Angelica oil	10
Costus oil	50
Sandalwood oil	100
Rose oil	25
Lavender oil	150
Bergamot oil	100
Paracresyl phenylacetate	25
Neroli	275
Amyl cinnamic aldehyde	100
C_9-C_{10}-aldehyde	10
C_{10}-C_{12}-aldehyde	15

Family of Sylvestriæ

Pine oil, mainly consisting of bornyl esters, is an example of a derivative from the Sylvestriæ which are akin to the lavenders in odour. Essences of forest pine, spruce, pumilio, etc., blend readily with lavender oils and yield with them very agreeable perfumes. Yet French perfumery has failed to make full use of Sylvestriæ odours, which deserve fuller attention than they have had.

Central Europe used to the full considerable quantities of birch shoots. These shoots yield a product which is unlike that from birch bark, a bark from which Russian leather perfumes are taken. Essences of pine shoots and needles are used in the main for hair lotions. Essence of oak moss has been used in the fern essence, which contains similar amounts of the sylvestrian and lavender derivatives of the former class. Chypre possesses a sylvestrian odour, whereas its odour was earlier regarded as that of a balsam. A chapter is devoted to chypre odours (see pp. 100-103).

Chypre Variety

Chypre I	*Grammes*
Essence of oak moss evernia	50
Bergamot oil	225
Vetiver oil (Bourbon)	75
Oil of lavender (in solvents)	50
Sandalwood oil or Indochina cedar oil	70
Patchouli oil	10
Essence of cloves (extra)	35
Essence of jasmine complex	100
Essence of rose complex	80
Isobutyl salicylate	70
Cinnamic storax alcohol	50
Heliotropin	100
Coumarin	50
Resinaroma of tonka bean	20
Methyl nonyl acetic aldehyde to C_{10}	15

American Dentifrice VIII

	Grammes
Essence of mint (Provençal)	350
Coriander oil	150
Anise oil	100
Chinese anise oil	150
Wintergreen oil	50
Essence of tarragon	25
Sweet orange oil	50
Menthol	75

Terpeneless Essence for Dentifrice IX

	Grammes
Mint (French, terpeneless)	500
Anise (Spanish, terpeneless)	400
Cinnamon oil (Ceylon, terpeneless)	30
Clove oil	30
Rose oil free from stearoptene (French)	40

Essence for Dentifrice X

	Grammes
Menthol (crystalline)	550
Anethol (crystalline)	400
Cinnamic aldehyde	20
Eugenol	20
Thymol or carvacrol	10

The proportions can be considerably varied. Spice essences such as those of ginger, tarragon, pepper, nutmeg, celery, caramus and caraway can also be added. Really original, very pleasant tasting flavours are thus obtained.

Amber Family

There is a great demand for amber fragrances. But it can be said that these amber fragrances resemble only distantly that of ambergris with its indefinable tone. The leaning today is towards full bodied heavy clinging aromas, and the introduction of artificial musk has dealt a mortal blow to the natural amber fragrances.

Synthetic fixers should be employed instead of natural products such as civet, castoreum, musk, tonkin or even Resinodour Labdanum.

Substances which are chemically identical to or related to the ambers and natural musks—*e.g.*, civettone, muscone or exaltone—generally have the true notes of the fixatives used by our grandparents.

While the nitro-musks are used in some recipes of this book, they are only used with reluctance and with a desire to be modern.

Nitrated musks should not be used at all, or, if used, then only in minimum quantities in quality products; further, they should be used with natural resinous fixatives such as infusions of natural musk, civet, castoreum or amber, and in the case of very high quality products with the substitutes discovered by Ruzicka.

Here is an up-to-date recipe based on synthetic nitrated musk.

Musk Variety

Musk for Extract I

	Grammes
Musk ketone	70
Musk ambrette	20
Resinodour benzoin	20
Resinodour labdanum	100
Resinodour ambrette	20
Resinodour tolu balsam	25
Sandalwood oil	80
Essence of rose complex	280
Bergamot oil	255
Isobutyl salicylate	40
Crystalline heliotropin	90

Musk Composition for Extract II

	Grammes
Musk ketone	70
Artificial amber in pieces	30
Musk ambrette	20
Sandalwood oil	80
Bergamot oil	100
Clary sage oil	50
Rose absolute oil	20
Artificial red rose	260
Isobutyl salicylate	100
Heliotropin	90
Rhodinol	95
α-Ionone	85

Liquid Musk for Extract III

	Grammes
Infusion of natural musk (20 per cent.)	150
Infusion of ambergris	150
Musk ketone	60
Musk ambrette	20
Artificial red rose	240
Patchouli oil	40
Bergamot oil	40
Sandalwood oil	20
Absolute jasmine oil	30
French geranium oil	45
Methyl ionone	40
Resinodour labdanum	100
Phenylethy lalcohol	35
Clary sage oil	30

Amber Variety

	Grammes
Resinodour labdanum	350
Resinodour vanilla	150
Resinodour tonka	85
Resinodour tolu balsam	100
Civet absolute	40
Castoreum absolute	50
Musk tonkin	40
Civettone synthetic	25
Sandalwood oil	80
Rose absolute oil	50
Jasmine absolute	30

Tincture of natural ambergris, tinctures of musks and civet can be used in place of the corresponding absolutes.

Fouquet recommends the addition of C_8 and C_9 aldehydes to up-to-date amber perfumes in order to increase the pronounced effect of the completed extract.

Old Amber for Extract II

	Grammes
Tincture of ambergris (20 per cent.)	85
Essence of rose composition	320
Vanillin	50
Heliotropin	150
Musk ketone	40
Musk ambrette	30
α-Ionone	125
Sandalwood oil	25
Essence of jasmine complex	25
Artificial cinnamic alcohol	150

Amber for Extract III

	Grammes
Resinodour Labdanum	45
Artificial amber	175
Tincture of ambergris (20 per cent.)	155
Methyl ionone	75
Rose oil composition	155
Jasmine absolute oil	10
Vetiver oil (Bourbon)	30
Clary sage oil	25
Resinodour benzoin	175
Vanillin	15
Heliotropin	50
Musk ketone	60
Musk ambrette	30

Use of Artificial Perfumes

Artificial (synthetic) perfume materials play the same part in formulations as essential oils, absolutes or balsams. If it is desired to prepare a lotion or an extract with the fragrance corresponding to that of an artificial perfume, it is not enough simply to dissolve 100 grammes for an extract, or 20 grammes for a lotion, in a litre of alcohol.

An alcoholic perfume should convey to the olfactory sense the following sensations by degrees: first, the perception of light fruity fragrances blended with the odour of alcohol; second, the stronger and more alcoholic floral odours; and finally, the heavy slightly volatile tones, subdued but persistent, or the basic odours of fixatives.

Therefore in making 100 grammes of the complete formulation for use either as an extract or as a lotion the following quantities of ingredients are used: 10-20 grammes of a complex of orange-like or other suitable fruit essence with its characteristic fragrance, 60-70 grammes of a mixture containing a more or less large proportion of artificial products and natural products, and 5-20 grammes of fixatives such as matured tinctures of musk, amber, civet, castoreum, resinodours and balsams or synthetic fixatives.

These various products are dissolved in alcohol and the solution is allowed to mature for as long a period as possible, although it may be noted that the process can be accelerated by "cleavage." The matured extract is chilled and finally filtered at low temperature in order to avoid the possibility of pitching in the winter.

PART II

ALCOHOLIC PERFUMES

Pride of place among alcoholic perfumes belongs to what were earlier termed scented waters, a description applied to the distillates of mixed plants, flowers or odoriferous seeds in spirit. It can be appreciated that such preparations were hardly likely to have a powerful aroma and that they would not bear comparison with modern products.

Gradually, as manufacturers brought essential oils—quintessences—into use they found themselves able to prepare still stronger solutions in alcohol. They therefore adopted distinctions between extracts, waters, and alcoholic perfumes.

These latter are the prototypes of hygiene helps which everyone has the right to use daily. They should be used daily by the woman who finds certain toilet refinements necessary, by the man as a cosmetic for his face and hair, and by the child, a flower in itself, and whose delightful aroma must not be spoiled by that of stale food. These are inherent to all civilised beings, the present-day ideas of those social reformers who desire to make us shed some of our customs rather than help to bring such good habits within reach of the humblest. Each worker desires the refinements and elegances to which his wealthier contemporaries are accustomed. Why should he not enjoy the perfumed articles of hygiene?

The exchequer seeks to perpetuate this inequality.

Toilet waters, less expensive than extracts, should be reasonably priced products. Despite the duties payable on alcohol, it can be used as the base for excellent products at a reasonable price.

The first chapter will deal with Colognes and with fancy toilet waters, incorrectly described as floral Colognes; lavender waters, their properties and their uses, particularly among sportsmen, will be discussed; lastly, handkerchief perfumes. Attention will be drawn to the "happy medium," drawn in commerce, between these extremes.

I. TOILET WATERS

Eau-de-Cologne

Alcoholic lotions having a variety of odours are described as and sold under the term Eaux-de-Cologne. This mistaken description becomes, in course of time, accepted. But the manufacturer should know the origin of the misnomer.

True eaux-de-Cologne are those products which reached the zenith of perfection a century ago. They can be improved only if some of their original qualities are sacrificed. It is essential that a manufacturer before creating a "Cologne water firm" should be well informed of the classical traditions on which such a water is based and, furthermore, that he should only depart from them with discretion and moderation.

Some formulæ have to be considered which are or might be thought obsolete. But they must be kept in mind.

The lemon-perfumed composition of the French Pharmacopœia is interesting. Its formula is:

Lemon Perfumed Alcohol

	Grammes
Lemon oil	4
Bergamot oil	4
Cedrat oil	4
Rosemary	4
Neroli	2
Lavender oil	2
Cinnamon oil	1
Alcohol solution of meliss balm	60
Alcohol	600

Leave to stand for 4 days and then distil four-fifths.

This pleasant, fresh, lively product deserves to be rated as a model among reference samples.

The *Perfumer Journal,* after an investigation of Farina's original formula, suggests:

	Grammes
Bulgarian rose oil	2
Jasmine oil	40
Geranium oil (Spanish)	40
Neroli	120
Lavender oil	40
Rosemary	10
Petitgrain oil (French)	120
Bergamot oil	240

for 36 litres of 94° alcohol and 4 litres of orange flower water. This quantity corresponds to 16 grammes of essential oils per litre.

A second but somewhat simplified formula is:

	Grammes
Neroli	100
Bergamot oil	220
Petitgrain oil	120
Lemon oil	180
Geranium oil	40
Rose oil	4
Lavender oil	40
Jasmine oil	8

for 100 litres of alcohol.

A modern formula for comparison is:

	Grammes
Bergamot oil	100
Linalyl acetate	250
Lemon oil	200
Citral distilled from lemon	62
Artificial neroli	120
Essence of Portugal	50
Lavender oil	50
Terpineol	30
Petitgrain oil	30
Rosemary	30
Artificial rose	20
Vanillin	20
Eugenol	10
Ethyl cinnamate	10
Resinodour labdanum	10
Resinodour benzoin	10

This is a slightly amber coloured, fixed Cologne water.

The following are classical formulæ:

Eau-de-Cologne I

	Grammes
Neroli	870
Rosemary	560
Lemon oil	250
Lemon petitgrain oil	100
Essence of Portugal	200
Oil of sweet lime	210
Bergamot oil	400
Rosewood oil	50
Benzyl acetate	10
Citral distilled from lemon	200

Eau-de-Cologne II

	Grammes
Bergamot oil	300
Lemon oil	300
Bitter orange oil	500
Oil of sweet lime	100
Petitgrain oil (terpeneless)	400
Orange ketone	40
Aurantiax	40
Terpenyl acetate	500
Citral distilled from lemon	310

In both these formulæ 5-10 grammes per litre of alcohol according to strength. The odour of orange flower is pronounced in each.

René Cerbelaud's work on Benedictine and his acute faculty of smell must be greatly admired. He would have been a great perfumer if he had not played with the thousands of rough formulæ he drew up. Here is one of his formulæ:

	Grammes
Bergamot oil	6
Lemon oil	6
Oil of cedrat	0·4
Clove oil	0·1
Lavender oil	1
Petitgrain oil	0·1
Rosemary	1
Red thyme	1
Saturated solution of artificial musk	5
Solution of rhodinol (to 10)	0·6
Tincture of benzoin (to 5)	10
Orange flower water	10
Rose water	40
Alcohol 90°	850
Distilled water	150

He recommends a drop of œnanthic ether per 10 litres of preparation so as to imitate the odour of wine alcohol.

One must admire the manufacturers' desires to maintain both the traditions and classical nature of the recipes.

The perfumer, however, seeks to go further. He superimposes floral fragrances on the essential Cologne odour and such developments lead to formulæ in which the main issue is obscured. There are recipes—for example, a violet extract—which do not contain the characteristic ingredients. They do, however, have many ingredients which, unwittingly, have in combination the desired aroma.

Felix Cola (*Le Livre du Parfumeur*) gives:

Floral Cologne Water (Eau-de-Cologne)

	Grammes
Neroli petals	30
Orange flower absolute	20
Bergamot	210
Lemon	210
Lavender	50
Rosemary	30
White thyme	20
Bulgarian rose	10
Jasmine absolute	10
Hydroxycitronellal	80
Concrete orris	5
Methyl ionone	65
Heliotropin	70
Clary sage	10
Hyssop	30
Angelica	5
Petitgrain	50
Nerol	95

While the preparation is well balanced, it is questionable whether it can be said to relate to an eau-de-Cologne. A distinction can be drawn between the constituents of the original formula and those of a violet/lilac composition. While the latter has its charm, it overweighs the former.

There are now two classes of floral eaux-de-Cologne. The first comprises those waters which maintain their hesperidin-like essence content or those which are mixtures of Cologne and floral waters; the second class have nothing in common with eaux-de-Cologne, and are lotions of either the flowers of the world or fancy fashionable perfumes.

This, of course, does not exclude the "botanical" mixtures and the essential oils obtained from herbs provided they have a nice aroma.

Cola's No. 4 is:

	Grammes
Bergamot	300
Lemon	370
Lavender	80
Hyssop	10
Marjoram	10
Carvone	10
Cardamom	10
Ceylon cinnamon	10
Clove	20
Wild thyme	15
Angelica	5
Tarragon	5
Balm mint	30
White thyme	25
Benzoin resinodour	65

Take out the benzoin, add some sugar and you have a kind of Benedictine!

It must be admitted that the old technique is not assisted by the veritable modern storehouse of varied new chemically synthesised ingredients. Such variations as are desired must be carefully sought.

A distinctly modern note can be given to Colognes by subtly adjusted aldehyde combinations. But care is necessary for it. It is claimed that such an addition will not interfere with the hygienic value of the divine balm.

Russian and Amber-like Cologne Waters (*Eaux-de-Cologne*)

Formularies still give recipes in which synthetic musks, such as xylene, ketone or ambrette musks, appear together with vanillin or coumarin.

Felix Cola uses these products freely in his so-called Russian formula and perhaps a little less freely in his amber odour formula.

Amber Cologne

	Grammes
Bergamot	300
Lemon	300
Lavender	40
Rosemary	20
Neroli	20
White thyme	20
Petitgrain	40
Heliotropin	100
Vanillin	30
Musk ambrette	40
Phenylethyl alcohol	30
Bulgarian rose	5
α-Ionone	45
Ambroin absolute	10

Russian Cologne

	Grammes
Bergamot	260
Lemon	280
Lavender	60
Rosemary	40
Linalyl acetate	30
α-Ionone	100
Neroli petals	20
Iso-eugenol	50
Musk ketone	30
Musk ambrette	20
Coumarin	10
Vanillin	40
Heliotropin	60

It is lack of imagination when coumarin is used in what is an essentially fresh preparation, for coumarin accentuates the odour of cut grass and dry herbs. Resins are better and they were formerly used.

Riess recommended tinctures of benzoin, orris and ambrette, others Tolu and Peru balsams, incense, opoponax, or gum resins. These tinctures do heighten and make more pleasant morning cleaning preparations.

It is most desirable to use a minimum of natural amber—today as dear as gold bullion—to give Cologne water an amber-like fragrance. So an amber-scented extract is used, an extract which our forebears named muscatel, after the wine, the taste of which was not unlike the aroma of the extract.

Vegetable bases used include clary or clary sage, angelica, resinodour or oil of labdanum, extract of saffron, resinodour of ambrette, mace, Tolu balsam, Tonka bean, vanilla, oil of celery, oak moss (provided it is used with caution), and essence of Daucus, which is more suitable for our purpose and has a more amber-like aroma than the oils of caraway, coriander, anise and fennel. Sometimes oil of visnage is used. It is considered that it is undesirable to use patchouli, sandalwood and vetiver in other than emergency cases in compositions with the fundamentally sweet odour of amber.

Among the animal bases are amber, musk, civet and castoreum. Their tinctures can be readily used, in particular that of civet. Civettone, muskone and Ruzicka's exaltone are not reproductions; they are the synthetic elements of these natural fixatives.

With some assiduity the manufacturer will be able to reproduce an amber perfume suitable for eau-de-Cologne and many other products. He thus reduces the use of nitrated musks to a minimum and seeks also to mask the odour, *sui generis*, since it can become unbearable in the course of time to a person who dislikes it.

There is no difficulty in compounding a spicy aroma, particularly as the supplies of the necessary materials are plentiful. Clove, which is not as a rule used alone, can be modified by various cinnamons, nutmeg, ginger, tarragon, cumin, thyme, peppers, pimentos, juniper, laurel, celery, bay, and cardamom. A carnation perfume is easy to formulate and too easy to find; so a strong and persistent blend of bases is sought so as to be more lively than the amber accompaniment. The amber can be a little too much "violoncello" even if the "contra-bass" is needed.

Mann and Winter, the Austrian perfumers, have similar opinions, although they do defer to the taste of chemists.

Russian Cologne	*Grammes*
Bergamot oil	40
Lemon oil	20
Essence of Portugal	20
Rosemary	4
Lavender oil	6
Oil of tangerine	2
Clove oil	2
Artificial neroli	12
Methyl ionone	0·5
Oak moss	0·5
Vanillin	5
Tincture of vanillin	150
Tincture of tolu balsam	250
Tincture of castoreum	35
Musk ambrette	20
Reconstituted amber	10
Ambrene	5

Too much oak moss leads to a chypre-like eau-de-Cologne. The addition of coumarin gives a note of cut grass, or fern, as it is termed today. Neither modification is regarded as unpleasant; but for the traditionalist distortions are to be found, and they but serve to satisfy the whims of buyers who are anything but judges of eaux-de-Cologne. Still, what does it matter, provided the buyer is satisfied?

The Use of Terpeneless Essential Oils

The increase of duties on alcohol used in perfumery coincided with Haensel's (Pirna) discovery of terpeneless oils. The manufacturers rapidly appreciated the advantages these new products possessed.

Louis Gattefossé, of Lyons, advanced their use in France and even carried out the arrangements to ensure the treatment of French essential oils to render them terpene-free. In the years since 1894 he has brought the terpene-free compositions for use in Cologne water to perfection.

To obtain a suitable perfume some 20-25 grammes of essential oils are needed, on an average, for each litre of 80° alcohol, and in Cologne preparations the terpene essences are very important. The finest expressed lemon oil contains 30-45 grammes of citrus aldehydes; the commercial oils 25-35 grammes per kilogramme, on the average. Haensel estimates that terpene-free lemon oil is some thirty times as concentrated as the expressed oil. More accurately it should be said that 30 kilogrammes of expressed oil are needed to yield 1 kilogramme of terpene-free oil. However, Haensel's statement is correct when the oils are used in juices and carbonated drinks, for their aroma is entirely due to the aldehydes.

It must be admitted that the terpenes have a fresh though somewhat weak odour. The systematic use of terpeneless lemon oil does not reproduce the fruit odour as accurately as does the oil-containing terpenes.

Similar comments are applicable to essence of Portugal—60 to 70 kilogrammes of this oil are necessary to obtain 1 kilogramme of terpene-free essence—and to tangerine oil, sweet lime, citron oil, etc.

Bergamot oil, on the other hand, contains some 50 per cent. of its weight of a terpene with a fine but weak odour. Other essences used in the preparation of eau-de-Cologne contain between 10 and 50 per cent. (rosemary) or 15 to 50 per cent. (lavender). Some French thymes contain 60 per cent. or more of terpenes, neroli 15 to 20 per cent. and pure petitgrain oil somewhat less. It will be seen that Haensel's calculation of concentration is not a reliable guide in the matching of perfumes.

Dorvault's formula for a lemon oil composition can be set out as follows:

	With essential oils Grammes	*With terpene free oils* Grammes
Lemon oil	400	20
Bergamot oil	400	180
Essence of cedrat	400	20
Rosemary oil	200	100
Neroli	200	150
Lavender oil	200	180
Cinnamon oil	100	80
Total	1,900	730

Thus the terpene-free mixture is some two and a half times as concentrated as the mixture of oils containing terpenes, so that 10 grammes of the former mixture against 25 grammes of the latter are necessary; 8 grammes suffice to replace the 20 grammes of the terpene-containing oils.

Alcohol 60° G.L. can be used in place of the 80° hitherto used. The odour of alcohol, particularly if it is wine alcohol, is strong and effective, but as the alcohol decreases in strength so does the odour. Thus, while 20 grammes of oils containing terpenes are needed in alcohol of 80°, only 5 grammes are needed for alcohol of 60° and 3 grammes for alcohol of 45° in the case of terpeneless oils.

The terpenes can be used in many products in which their solubility in alcohol is not of primary importance and in which volatile oils are desirable—*e.g.*, soap perfumes. In such perfumes both heavy and light components are used. The former are usually not used unless they contain terpenes, either because they are coloured and contain only slightly soluble polymers or because their fragrance is not sufficiently fine.

The terpene-free oils are not as expensive as their concentration might suggest. In fact, when all aspects are taken into consideration, terpene-free oils offer many advantages.

But it might well be asked, Do not the double or triple rectified oils give just as good results?

Essential oils intended for use in fine perfumes are sometimes rectified by steam distillation. The stills used have a long swan-neck which allows a fairly good fractionation to be obtained. During each distillation some 10 per cent. initial fractions and 10-15 per cent. of the final fractions are put aside, the amounts being dependent on the age of the product being distilled. Polymerisation can occur fairly rapidly with oils containing terpenes and possibly traces of water from the steam distillation process, and the oils thus come to contain sesquiterpenes. A four-year-old oil of lavender can lose 15 to 20 per cent. of its weight, and an oil of mint up to 35 per cent., and still contain terpenes.

Lemon and orange oils change rapidly and the polymers have an unpleasant odour, so that steam distillation is next to useless. The oils cannot be used.

The use of anhydrous, terpene-free oils is interesting, for the oils will not deteriorate on storage. They will not oxidise in the absence of terpenes and water, and therefore there will be no losses due to storage.

These advantages are so much in favour of the process of eliminating terpenes from oils that the process has been universally adopted by perfumery manufacturers.

The manufacturer who has no interest except in the good finish of his products and leaves supplies to his manager is only interested in some of his products. For the manufacturer there is the problem as to whether terpene-free oils will give him products equally as good as oils with terpenes.

By following the development of different formulations the problem may be answered.

Cerbelaud quotes the following formula:

	C.c.
Distilled orange flower water	10
Distilled rose water	40
Distilled water	150
Alcohol 90°..	800
Bergamot oil	6
Lemon oil	6
Cedrat oil	0·4
Clove oil	0·1
Lavender oil	1
Petitgrain oil	1
Thyme oil	1
Saturated solution of artificial musk ..	5
Solution of rhodinol (to 10)	0·6
Tincture of benzoin (to 5)	10

When the formula is recalculated on the basis of 100 litres, 0·25 gramme neroli water can be regarded as equivalent to 1 litre orange flower water and 1 gramme of stearoptene-free rose essence to rose water. The musk solution contains 2·5 grammes, the rhodinol solution about 6 grammes of rhodinol, and the tincture of benzoin about 200 grammes of resinodours.

The formula calculated on the basis of terpene-free pure ingredients is:

	Grammes
Bergamot oil (terpene-free)	270
Lemon oil (terpene-free)	40
Cedrat oil (terpene-free)	2
Clove oil (terpene-free)	8
Lavender oil (terpene-free)	90
Petitgrain oil (terpene-free)	9
Rosemary oil (terpene-free)	50
Thyme oil (terpene-free)	35
Rhodinol	6
Artificial musk	2·5
Benzoin resinodour	200
Neroli water	0·5
Stearoptene-free rose	1

It can be seen that the formula specifies too much rosemary and thyme and too little petitgrain and neroli; the other ingredients are a matter of individual taste.

The essences used are 500 grammes per 100 litres as opposed to 1,560 grammes when terpene-containing oils are used.

The new formula can be used with a lower grade of alcohol and, if this course is followed, 4 grammes or even less can be used per litre of alcohol.

Although the result is not the same exactly, the odour similarity is extraordinarily close. From a physiological point of view the rubefacient action of the terpenes is reduced. Here attention must be drawn to a fault the purveyors of eau-de-Cologne perpetrate. If the preparation is made up in 60° alcohol, the tonic and counter-irritant properties are inferior to those of an eau-de-Cologne made up with 80° alcohol; the sellers should not offer the articles in 60° alcohol as frictions. Yet waters with 60° or 70° alcohol can be made so as to have a delicate yet concentrated fragrance.

It has been found by experience that the solubility of the mixtures is directly proportional to the solubility of their constituents.

For example, lemon oils are soluble in 80° alcohol in a ratio of 1 : 30, whereas terpeneless essences are soluble to the same extent in 60° alcohol. A mixture of 18 parts terpene-free and 2 parts terpene-containing oils is soluble in 62° alcohol; a 15:5 mixture in 65° alcohol; a 10 : 10 mixture in 75° alcohol. It is thus easy to use proportionate amounts of the terpene oils, within the required solubility limits, by varying the alcohol used.

The strength of the alcohol can be reduced by decreasing the amounts of oils used. The terpene-free oil is soluble in alcohol of 45° to an amount of 5 grammes per litre. With just the minimum of filtration—for brilliancy—and with a minimum of handling and of losses a commercial product with the original properties of the traditional formula is obtained.

Today, terpene-free essences are more essential than ever before. The present-day tax laws have raised the price of alcohol, and since prices of products are high, their quality must be high. Buyers, however, are not interested in the alcohol used; they demand, however, perfumes of first-rate quality in return for the high prices.

Cheap Eaux-de-Cologne

Competition frequently leads to a lowering of quality standards. Under the description of "Cheap Eaux-de-Cologne" are offered alcoholic solutions of various terpenes and synthetic perfumes. The least that can be said about these products is that they give the consumer a very poor idea of the professional conscience of certain traders who are undeserving of the name of perfumers.

The high cost of alcohol bars the use of low quality products in it. It is surely better to use but small amounts of a normally priced aromatic mixture than large amounts of a common composition.

Supplies at present on the market make it practicable for the conscientious manufacturer to make suitable formulations from the cheapest ingredients. These formulations should be soluble in the alcohol used so as to avoid the need for filtration, which is a source of losses. To arrive at the final strength a determination can be made with 60° alcohol, at a concentration of 5 grammes per litre, of the essences suitably made up with terpene-containing oils, terpene-free oils and artificial products. It is hardly necessary, in such determination, to exceed 33 per cent. for oils with terpenes—*e.g.*, lemon and orange. The other oils need only contain the minimum of terpenes.

Bergamot oil, usually containing some 50 per cent. terpenes, can be replaced by a synthetic terpene-free mixture made up of linalyl and terpenyl acetates and a small amount of neroli. Natural neroli is preferably replaced by a good petitgrain oil, rather than by complexes, the orange odour of which is due to synthetic methyl anthranilate.

Clearly it is a very powerful cheap substitute, but it is essential to know how to use it to the best advantage. Otherwise it can make the mixture not only insipid but sickening.

Mann and Winter (*Die Moderne Parfumerie*) give a formula of this nature:

Synthetic bergamot	300	grammes
Lemon oil	200	,,
Artificial neroli	100	,,
Lavender oil	50	,,
Petitgrain oil	20	,,
Rosemary	50	,,
Citral	5	,,
Methyl anthranilate	10	,,
Orange flower water	3	litres
Alcohol	30	,,

It will be seen that citral is used with discretion so as to avoid the odour of verbena, which is not pleasing, and that orange oil is absent. On the other side of the Rhine a fresh lemon odour is generally preferred to the hot odour of orange. The amount of methyl anthranilate is more than sufficient. While the quantity of 24 grammes per litre is used in the formula, it could be reduced to 7 to 8 grammes with advantages in respect both of cost and odour.

The following is a formula recommended by the Roret (Pradal, Malepeyre and Villon)—it is cheap:

	Grammes
Terpenyl acetate	300
Linalyl acetate	200
Geranyl acetate	50
Geraniol	50
Neroline	25
Ethyl phenacetate	10
Linalol	80
Terpineol	100
Citral	40
Piperonal	4

for 40 litres of alcohol.

It is certainly not astonishing that there are Cologne waters with not the slightest semblance of the aroma of the true commercial product. Despite the fact that the formula is mainly recommended for export, as the manual indicates, it is hoped that it will not be given a second trial by foreign manufacturers.

Floral Colognes

Is it essential to accept the market's tendency to sell eaux-de-Cologne which are floral toilet waters in reality? The question is difficult to answer, for in the long run the clientele commands and the manufacturer obeys. Even Empress Eugenie's perfumer appreciated a similar position. She expressed a desire for an Imperial water with the fragrances of a mixed flower garden. The Empress, however, did not ask for hesperidium-like essences.

There are few handkerchief perfumes which do not contain some proportion of volatile, light fresh base odours derived from hesperidium oils, strengthened with a good neroli. The different odours, together with that of the volatile alcohol, are necessary for the rounding off.

If a handkerchief preparation, standard at 15 per cent. of the absolute product, can only contain 3-5 per cent. of the key notes, a toilet water, standard at 30 per cent., will be able to have more.

Special compositions are necessary today for toilet waters. From the artistic viewpoint this may be far from the truth, from the technical position it is vital. There need be no special attention paid to the desirability of using either 70° or 75° alcohol, for 90° alcohol is always used. At this latter strength there is no difficulty in dissolving perfumery materials.

But at 75° or below this is not so, more especially when due allowance is made for variations in the "apparent degree" (see chapter on Filtration). The products can be subjected to temperatures as low as - 10° in showcases and, exceptionally, even - 20° during transit in winter, and hence a proper safety margin must be established.

Cerbelaud gives some formulæ for floral eaux-de-Cologne. He takes care to stress that 90° alcohol should be used, but this grade of alcohol is far too expensive for competition, and contains too much spirit for daily use in body and hair frictions.

The following is a floral (mimosa) Cologne 90°:

	Grammes
Bergamot oil	5
Lemon oil	12
Orange oil (Portugal)	10
Petitgrain oil	2
Lavender oil	1
Rosemary	0·5
White thyme oil	0·5
Neroli	1
Synthetic mimosa	2
Ylang-ylang	1
Para-methyl acetophenone	2
Cherry-kernel oil	0·1
α-Ionone	1
Benzyl acetate	0·25
Jasmine absolute	0·20
Musk ambrette	0·25
Tincture of resinodour compound	5

per 1 litre of rice alcohol 90°.

The formula is made up of a Cologne essence and a mimosa extract:

	Grammes
Essence for eau-de-Cologne	32
Mimosa composition	12

(See chapters on Eau-de-Cologne and Mimosa preparations.)

The essential problem has been left untouched—namely, to prepare a solution in either 75° or 80° alcohol so as to contain a minimum of 3 per cent. concentrate and to remain clear at very low temperatures.

There is a similar problem in the perfuming of a brilliantine made up of petroleum oil. Some perfumes are soluble in the oil, others are insoluble.

Essential oils, even terpeneless, differ in their solubility in dilute alcohol as the following table shows:

	Grams per litre	
	60° Alcohol	*70° Alcohol*
Angelica	5	25
Anise	5	25
Celery	2	5
Citronella grass	3	20
Lemon	5	35
Tarragon	7	15
Tangerine	2	15
Orange	2	30
Pine	2	15
Sandalwood	5	200
Vetiver	6	100
Ylang-ylang	8	40
Rosewood	150	600

Similar variations are met with in synthetics, artificial perfumes and their components. Alcohols and phenols are very soluble, sesquiterpenes are almost or wholly insoluble. As regards esters derived from an acid with different homologous alcohols, it is found that the solubility decreases as the molecular weight increases. With mixtures of alcohols and esters, the lower the ester content the more soluble is the mixture. For weak alcoholic lotions a 28° rather than 40° lavender ester is to be preferred.

Synthetic musks are generally only slightly soluble; coumarin is only slightly soluble; yara and neroline are weakly soluble; amyl salicylate causes trouble. Perfumes can be made almost, or completely, insoluble by accidental or intended additions of ethyl phthalate as a diluent. The manufacturing technique for artificial flower essences for use in lotions, toilet waters, and floral eaux-de-Cologne is purely a matter of trial and error. The subject has been carefully studied by some chemists and the reader is recommended to get into touch with them for compositions, concentrations for use, etc.

Hawthorn Eau-de-Cologne

	Grammes
Anisaldehyde	200
Crystalline coumarin	20
Liquid jasmine	30
Tincture of vanilla, resinodour	300
Tincture of tolu, resinodour	100
Tincture of musk	50

10 grammes per litre of alcohol and 2 grammes for Eau de Cologne.

Four Flower Cologne

	Grammes
Artificial musk	150
Artificial rose	300
Artificial jasmine	150
Artificial violet	100
Coumarin	50
Amorphous heliotropin	10
Methyl ionone	50
C_9-aldehyde	1
Natural jasmine absolute	20
Rose absolute	20
Orange flower absolute	15
Tincture of benzoin	100
Tincture of castoreum	35

10 grammes per litre of alcohol.

Cyclamen Cologne

	Grammes
Linalol (likari)	250
Terpineol	500
Hydroxycitronellal	50
Methyl ionone	75
Artificial lily of the valley	75
Nonyl aldehyde	2·5
Jasmin absolute	7·5

Instructions as before

Coreopsis Cologne

	Grammes
Artificial red rose	100
Lilac base X	100
Artificial honeysuckle	100
Artificial cyclamen	100
Artificial amber (in pieces)	125
Artificial salvia	420
Petitgrain oil (Paraguaya, terpeneless)	10
Artificial jasmine	45

10 grammes per litre of alcohol.

Fern Cologne

	Grammes
Bergamot oil (terpeneless)	400
Coumarin	300
Absolute essence of green lavender	100
Geranium oil (Algiers, terpeneless)	40
Artificial carnation	60
Tincture of artificial amber	200
Artificial violet	92
Oak moss, Evernia	8

Instructions as for preceding.

Lily Cologne

	Grammes
Artificial broom	250
Coumarin	250
Artificial mock orange	250
Artificial heather	125
Hydroxycitronellal	100
Lily absolute	25

The same instructions as above.

Gardenia Cologne

	Grammes
Vanillin	40
Benzyl acetate	50
Artificial tuberose	100
Artificial mimosa	50
Ionone	5
Artificial rose	20
Clover (100 per cent.)	50
Benzyl hydroxyamyl	20
Tincture of musk	200
Tincture of tolu	200
Natural violet leaves	5
Orange flower absolute	5

The same instructions as above.

Broom Cologne

	Grammes
Terpineol	500
Isobutylphenylacetate	200
Methyl acetophenone	100
Hydroxycitronellal	100
Isoeugenol	10
Crystalline neroline	30
Artificial tuberose	50

The same instructions as above.

Glycine Cologne

	Grammes
Artificial lily of the valley	500
β-Ionone	125
New jasmine flowers	185
Methyl anthranilate	3
Artificial honeysuckle	125
Yara-yara	10
French labdanum resinodour	50
Jasmine absolute	5

The same instructions as above.

Heliotrope Cologne

	Grammes
Terpineol	450
Heliotropin	200
Vanillin	100
Musk ketone	50
Artificial jasmine	100
Methyl acetophenone	10
Petitgrain oil (terpeneless)	20
Oil of real bitter almonds	5
Neroli	25
Artificial tuberose	25

The same instructions as above.

Jonquil Cologne

	Grammes
Essence of rosewood (terpeneless)	50
Artificial mimosa	100
Artificial jonquil	50
Artificial narcissus	100
Phenyl acetic aldehyde	5
Hydroxycitronellal	75
Bromstyrol	20
Crystalline neroline	20
Amber (in pieces)	60
Hyacinth absolute	20
Tincture of benzoin	500

Instructions as above.

Narcissus Cologne

	Grammes
Terpineol	370
Brazilian rosewood (terpeneless)	150
Benzyl acetate	60
Paracresol	10
Vanillin ethyl derivative	10
Terpenyl acetate	250
Crystalline heliotropin	10
Geranium oil (terpeneless)	10
Phenylethyl alcohol	100
Paracresyl phenyl acetate	10
Musk ambrette	20

Instructions as above.

Carnation Cologne

	Grammes
Isoeugenol	100
Acetyl eugenol	100
Eugenol	100
Methyl isoeugenol	50
Terpineol	485
Geraniol	180
Benzyl acetate	100
Oil of lavender (terpeneless)	25
Crystalline heliotropin	40
Muskene	20
Yara-yara	10

Instructions as above.

Orchid Cologne

	Grammes
Amyl salicylate	300
Lavender oil (terpeneless)	10
Geranium oil (Algiers, terpeneless)	50
Isoeugenol	20
Terpineol	200
Linalol	200
Ylang-ylang	50
Artificial amber (in pieces)	50
Bromelia	20
Jasmine absolute	10

Same instructions as above.

Rose Cologne

	Grammes
Phenylethyl alcohol	70
Geranium of palmarosa	160
D-Citronellol	195
Linalol	80
Deltax base	20
Essence of guaiac wood	20
Geranium oil (Algiers, terpeneless)	250
Benzyl acetate	100
Rose absolute	50
C_9-aldehyde	1
Citral	1

Same instructions as above.

French Rose Cologne

	Grammes
Geraniol	500
Terpineol	180
Ionone	100
Geranium oil (Algiers, terpeneless)	75
Phenylethyl alcohol	75
Rhodinol	50
C_{10}-aldehyde	2
Amber (in pieces)	20

The same instructions as above.

Clover Cologne

	Grammes
Amyl salicylate	350
Linalyl acetate	80
Rosewood linalol	160
Terpineol	50
Essence of lavender water	75
Essence of green lavender absolute	25
Oak moss, Evernia	5
Crystalline heliotropin	25
Patchouli (terpeneless)	5
Sandalwood (terpeneless)	25
Vanillin	25
Methyl ionone	125
Musk xylene	40

The same instructions as above.

Verbena Cologne

	Grammes
Essence of French verbena	500
Artificial violet	150
Benzyl isoeugenol	20
Amber (in pieces)	30
Tincture of orris	100
Tincture of tolu resinodour	100
Tincture of ambrette resinodour	100

Instructions as above.

Violet Cologne

	Grammes
Artificial Parma violet	785
Artificial jasmine	40
Deltax base	10
Crystalline floranol	20
Amber (in pieces)	30
Resinodour of ambrette	30
Resinodour of cistus	25
Resinodour of orris	50
Absolute of violet leaves	10

The same instructions as above.

Eau-de-Cologne: Should the Cologne be Fixed?

There appears to be two schools of thought on this question among manufacturers. Some original eaux-de-Cologne are not fixed; they readily evaporate and leave no persistent odour. Others, particularly those of French manufacture and following the classical traditions, contain either benzoin or benzoin substitutes.

French perfumers, perforce, adopted a formula based on denatured alcohol and synthetic musk, and the national clientele has accordingly become accustomed to the dusty, musty smell which persists after application.

The French clientele actually prefers a tenacious perfume, despite the fact that it may be one that is superimposed on a real perfume. Eaux-de-Cologne are products which can be regarded as suitable for general use—on the train during a journey, maybe on holidays or even at home. Sometimes it is used at the wrong moment—*e.g.*, prior to the user being exposed to powerful sunlight on the mountain-side or on the seashore. Such uses, at the wrong time, may lead to sunstroke or to pronounced tan.

Because eau-de-Cologne is not considered to be a perfume it need not leave a characteristic odour. That floral toilet waters can leave some trace of their odour which can mingle with perfumes subsequently used is an argument against their general use. For this very reason perfume firms frequently market an extract, a toilet water and a face powder with the same perfume.

The solution to the problem is essentially a compromise. There need be no marked fixation except for amber Cologne. The very name suggests its tenacity. The recognisable odour of synthetic musk can be imparted by a mixture of musk and resin.

Mann and Winter (*Die Moderne Parfumerie*) give a recipe for a modern, fully fixed eau-de-Cologne:

	Grammes
Neroli, bitter orange	4
Petitgrain oil	1
Bergamot oil	10
Lemon oil	5
Portugal oil	5
Rosemary	2·5
Lavender	2·5
Tincture of benzoin	5
Tincture of musk	1
Tincture of orris	2
Bulgarian rose oil	0·1
Ylang-ylang	0·05

A further example is taken from the same work. It is for an amber-scented Cologne.

Amber-scented Imperial

(*For Eau-de-Cologne* 85°: 1½ *litres*)

	Grammes
Musk ambrette	6
Vanillin	4
Artificial amber	4
Ambrene	6
Tincture of castoreum	10
Tincture of vanilla	15
Tincture of tolu	25
Tincture of musk	15
Essence of labdanum	1·5
Oak moss absolute	0·3
Bulgarian rose oil	0·5

The fixative is roughly at least equal in quantity to that of the essential oils. This may be excessive in the opinion of French makers. An example is the addition of amber perfume to "base" odours, but the addition must be made with discretion. While the aroma of the finished product is somewhat heavy, as a French odour, it is nevertheless quite agreeable.

Imperial Lemery Water contained nutmeg, cinnamon, clove, calamus, sandalwood, laurel, hyssop, saw-wort, as well as other ingredients of eau-de-Cologne. Déjean (1787) stated that the predominant note should be laurel.

Felix Cola (*Le Livre du Parfumeur*) recommends only the following essence composition for a Russian eau-de-Cologne:

	Grammes
Bergamot oil	260
Lemon oil	280
Lavender	60
Rosemary	40
Neroli oil	20
Linalyl acetate	30
α-Ionone	100
Isoeugenol	50
Musk ketone	30
Musk ambrette	20
Coumarin	10
Vanillin	40
Heliotropin	60

This ultimately gives about 15 per cent. fixative in relation to the total weight and not 50 per cent. as in the German example.

It should be noted that the quantity of fixative is lower still for a simple amber-scented eau-de-Cologne.

	Grammes
Bergamot oil	300
Lemon oil	300
Lavender	40
Rosemary	20
Neroli oil	20
White thyme	20
Petitgrain oil	40
Bulgarian rose oil	5
α-Ionone	45
Phenylethyl alcohol	30
Heliotropin	100
Vanillin	30
Musk ambrette	40
Ambreine absolute	10

If it is assumed that heliotropin imparts the floral tone, then there is about 8 per cent. fixative; if it is assumed to be a fixative, there is about 18 per cent.

This amount is not excessive when it is recalled that other current eau-de-Cologne formulæ contain perhaps 5-7 per cent fixatives. They do sometimes contain none at all.

The examples illustrate that quite a wide variation occurs. In general French perfumers slightly fix their ordinary Colognes and strongly fix their amber or Russian Colognes.

Eau-de-Portugal

This is not wholly obsolete. Essentially it is an eau-de-Cologne in which the citrus elements are kept and lavender and rosemary omitted.

	Grammes
Terpeneless orange oil	5
Citral	3
Artificial neroli	3
C_{10}-aldehyde (to 10	5
Cologne fixative	5

for 1 litre of alcohol.

Oil of neroli (Portugal) with terpenes is only used when the alcohol strength is above 75°.

A fresher, lighter variation is:

Portugal II

	Grammes
Terpeneless bitter orange oil	7
Clementier (terpeneless)	5
Neroli oil (terpeneless)	2
Bergamot oil	3
Artificial musk	1

These formulæ can be varied by adding to them eau-de-Cologne compositions:

	Grammes
Sweet orange oil	5
Oil of clementier	5
Citral	3
Petitgrain oil	3
C_{10}-aldehyde (to 10)	5
Essence for Eau-de-Cologne	3
Fixative for Eau-de-Cologne	2

Eau-de-Quinine

This lotion is not found so frequently as it was in trade circles. It should contain quinine sulphate to merit its name, but of course the use of the salt should be left to a pharmacist. It is not for the perfumer.

	Grammes
Geranium oil (terpeneless)	10
Methyl ionone	5
Clove oil	3
Rose fixative	5

for 1 litre of alcohol.

Bay rum preparations should really contain some bay rum.

Bay Rum

	Grammes
Oil of bay	12
Bergamot oil	12
Spicy fixative	6

Lavender Waters and Spirits of Lavender

Lavender waters and spirits of lavender have been widely used in personal toilets and even in the washing of clothes. Their name is derived from that of the plant.

The straight lavender water was prepared by the distillation of a mixture of water and flowers; a similar process was used to prepare lavender spirits, but wine spirit was used instead of water.

The traditional colour of lavender water was red until a few years ago. The water contained, according to A. B. Lunel's (1870) *Practical Guide,* such ingredients as sage, hyssop, speedwell, rose of Provence, balm mint, artemesia, agrimony, absinthe, fennel and balsam.

Pradal, Malepeyre and Villon give the following basic formula for lavender spirit in their *Manuel du Parfumeur*:

Lavender (dry flowers)	3 kg. 125 grammes
Alcohol 85°	26 litres

Sufficient water is added so that on distillation 40 to 50 litres of about 40° spirit are obtained.

Old formularies are somewhat reserved on this subject. It is essential to read modern works to appreciate perfumery trends.

H. Mann (*Die Moderne Parfumerie*) gives:

	Grammes
Lavender essence	85
Lemon oil	10
Geranium oil	5
Peru balsam	32
Artificial amber	15
Musk tincture	50
Civet tincture	25
Storax tincture	150
Vanillin	10
Héliotropin	8

for 5 litres of alcohol.

The formula yields a lotion smelling of amber, balsam and dry lavender. The aroma is far removed from that which customers want, a fresh smell redolent of freshly gathered flowers.

The same author's formula for Royal Lavender water is the preceding one to which isoeugenol and cinnamon oil have been added. The betterment of the aroma is due to the orris tincture that is present in small amount.

Cerbelaud has for long devoted himself to the study of lavender waters. He soon realised that the true amateurs often prefer the simple lavender tinctures to the complex, amber-scented lavender waters. He both uses and abuses coumarin as well as β-methyl umbelliferone in his formulæ for new-mown grass perfumes. He recommends also the use of an alcoholic "truffle." This is an indication of his liking for lavender oils from the Apt region. These oils create an illusion of being in the neighbourhood of mushrooms.

Laying aside other considerations, which need not be repeated here, he states that "the lavender essences cannot be isolated from rose, bergamot and neroli oils (in small concentrations), nor from sweet-orange oils, tincture of orris (at somewhat higher concentrations), methyl ionone . . . clary sage still gives an excellent floral note." This agrees with the tastes of today's amateurs. He draws attention to obsolete and forgotten fixatives, recommends the use of labdanum tincture and that of exaltolide for the trio, amber-musk-civet.

Here is the recommended formula:

	Grammes
Fine lavender oil	20
Lavender absolute	1
Rosemary	0·5
Neroli oil	0·5
Geranium oil	0·5
Musk ketone	1
Tincture of benzoin to 10	4

for 1 litre of alcohol.

This formula should simulate Yardley's lavender, according to Cerbelaud, but the responsibility is his.

The following is a more complex formula:

Cerbelaud Lavender

	Grammes
Essence of lavender	27
Decolorised lavender absolute	2
Methylate of β-umbelliferone	0·5
Coumarin	0·2
Alpine rosemary	0·5
Neroli oil	0·75
Bergamot oil	0·5
Bulgarian rose oil	0·25
Tincture of mastic	5
Musk ketone	1
Crystalline exaltolide	0·1

for 1 litre of alcohol.

Variations contain methyl ionone, dianthax or dianthine, thyme oil or synthetic esters, replaced by linalyl acetate.

One of his amber formulæ must be quoted if only because the question of handkerchief perfumes will shortly be considered.

Amber-like Lavender Water

	Grammes
Lavender oil	25
Bergamot oil	10
Clary sage	1
Sandalwood oil	1
Infusion of orris	50
,, storax	40
,, tolu	5
,, Peru	3
,, ambergris	3
,, civet	2
,, musk	5

for 1 litre of alcohol mixed with rose water.

Cola speaks unemotionally of lavender. He gives the following composition:

Lavender Extra

	Grammes
Lavender oil	600
Bergamot oil	100
Lemon oil	50
Bulgarian rose oil	10
Geranium oil	40
Coumarin	50
Isoeugenol	10
Musk ambrette	40
Resinodour benzoin	100

and the following for—

Fancy Lavender

	Grammes
Lavender oil	400
Lemon oil	50
Patchouli oil	10
Citronellyl acetate	60
Geranyl acetate	100
Nerol	40
Coumarin	50
Vetiverol	20
Linalyl acetate	100
Linalyl propionate	30
Musk ambrette	20
Musk ketone	20
Heliotropin	90

It is primarily a matter of opinion as well as of composition for an original perfume like that of lavender. The subject will be referred to again in the following chapter. The floral odour that heliotropin gives should be kept in mind, particularly as the odour corresponds closely to that of fresh lavender spirit.

Fouquet gives in his *Technique Moderne* the following formula:

	Grammes
Lavender flower oil	300
Great lavender oil	50
Linalyl acetate	100
Infusion of natural vanilla	100
Infusion of musk ambrette	50
Musk xylene	20

for 9¼ litres alcohol and 275 c.c. rose water.

Provided that great lavender oil is a good and proper French oil, it will have its merits. It is appreciated particularly in the soap industry and sometimes in perfumery. It is forgotten too often, probably because of the lack of quality in the oils offered.

Thus, despite the indifference of perfumers towards lavender oil and its aroma, the various formulæ show the interest evinced in lavender, the aroma of dry flowers. This aroma is associated with the lavender bags used in linen cupboards. The English, who buy bunches of fresh flowers, have perhaps realised fuller and better the charms of the fine petals of the flowers.

Since its introduction the authors have recommended lavender oil to be used in volatile solvents. As there is a deepening appreciation by buyers it is desirable to determine whether the odour of dry herb or cut grass is over-stressed. This can be readily appreciated. Formerly the method of production of essential oils from lavender and lavandin profoundly affected their properties. Harvesting of the flowers should be carried out quickly. During the summer months there are but few days between the time when the flowers are at their best and that when the seed is ripe. The flowers should therefore be gathered rapidly and the flower stems stacked after they have been dried. The distillation can be carried out in due course. The ingredients that make up the dry flower bouquet are fortunately almost non-volatile, and so the essential oils have this dry flower character rather than that of the fresh flower. The flower stems can be distilled immediately after garnering.

By taking out the soluble elements with petroleum solvents—the elements include the coumarin derivatives formed during drying—there is obtained an extract with a strong dried herb bouquet.

The manufacturers have taken cognisance of the position. They market varieties of absolutes from which the coumarin components have been more or less taken. In the place of the coumarin materials complexes with a more fashionable note have been introduced, particularly fatty aldehydes. These materials are given decorative names and will be used to replace the absolutes at the appropriate time.

Many perfumers wish to produce spirits of lavender with the beautiful fragrance of fresh flowers. The term "spirits" distinguishes the products from lotions which contain 15 to 25 grammes essential oil per litre of alcohol, whereas the former contain as a rule some 40 to 60 grammes. Because of their higher oil content spirits are filled into more elegant while not luxurious bottles.

The note of freshly cut flowers is obtained with the addition of a complex of suitable hesperidium essences—*e.g.*, lemon, orange, bergamot, tangerine, cedrat, sweet lime, neroli, and heliotropin. The bouquet of the Provence wild rose needs thyme oils, hyssop, and rosemary oil (from Provence and not exotic). The floral strength is dependent on the quality of the oil and the oil must be chosen with great care. Just as a wine taster who has journeyed and made his "pilgrimage of the mountains" in order to know the products and trees, so ought the perfumer. The plants of Diois have an aroma of pippin apples and many attempts are made to simulate it; those of Luberon carry the scent of fox; while those of the low Alps, Maritime Alps, Vaucluse and Lot have the classical odours with nuances. These form the basis of the needs of traders. The oils they yield can be made stronger and more feminine in note with clary sage.

When fashionable lavender waters are analysed they are often found to contain a high amount of esters. This led to Cerbelaud's belief that synthetic linalyl and geranyl esters, acetates and butyrates should be added to the essential oil. There is a much simpler explanation. The manufacturers who introduced this device (but who did not disclose it to the authors) will not be angry with them for their indiscrete enquiry; truth leaks out sooner or later.

A few millilitres of glacial acetic acid are added to the alcoholic solution of lavender oil. Esterification of the linalol is rapid in the presence of the alcohol, the fresh fragrance is heightened, the solution maintains its acid *p*H, and the somewhat acid musty smell (not acrid) contributes to the lively note that is desired.

Now as to fixation.

It has been repeated again and again that, in the opinion of some customers as well as the authors, nitrated musks soften and subdue subtle spring bouquets and that their entire removal, in this case, is wrong. This opinion is a personal one and there is no compulsion to share it (Galup no longer has any authority). Similarly there is little inclination to use balsams and resins which strengthen the "dry herb" odour to that of the apothecary's herbs. Artificial ambers, with vanillin or tolu notes, impart to lavender spirits an unsatisfactory aroma of "Armenian paper." While the absolute of labdanum has some very desirable properties, there is an art in the choice of the right one. Some labdanum gums can be boiled, reboiled and partly caramelised. They no longer contain any essential oil, and of course their aroma is affected. When it is recalled that an absolute can be obtained by extracting the plant directly and without boiling water, it is no wonder that the results are so different. The gum rosin absolute of the Moroccan rock-rose is very good; in combination with clary sage it yields excellent results.

Glycols are to be found in some of Cerbelaud's formulæ. These weakly volatile materials can function as physical fixatives, but it is necessary to render them odourless by a double distillation.

Natural amber, musk and civet are only excluded by price. Civettone and exaltolide can likewise be used, provided their cost allows it. New substances such as umulene have been developed by chemists. They will be assessed on their useful properties.

Thus, on the basis of these instructions, the perfumer can produce spirits of lavender. These products are attractive to many men; even those of little developed countries would doubtless appeciate it: and certainly their wives. All in all, they compose a market which is well worth capturing.

English Recipes

The authors consider it desirable to give some formulæ from English books (*Perfumes, Cosmetics and Soaps*, Chapman and Hall, London), since British labelled lavender extracts find a considerable market in the countries of the world.

Lavender 1214
(according to W. A. Poucher)

	Grammes
English lavender oil	15
French lavender oil	5
Bergamot oil	10
Clary sage	1
Tincture of civet (3 per cent.)	4
Infusion of orris	5

For 1,000 alcohol.

Lavender 1215
(*after W. A. Poucher*)

	Grammes
English lavender oil	12
Montblanc lavender	4
Neroli oil	0·5
Bergamot oil	2
Sweet orange oil	1
Tincture of musk (3 per cent.)	5
Tincture of civet (3 per cent.)	5
Tincture of storax	3
Tincture of orris	2
Tincture of ambrette essence (10 per cent.)	2
Vanillin	1
Benzyl isoeugenol	0·5

for 1,000 alcohol.

Lavender Composition 1216
(*after W. A. Poucher*)

	Grammes
French lavender oil	600
Bergamot oil	250
Neroli oil	20
Red rose oil	10
Concrete orris	20
Oak moss	1
Patchouli oil	1
Coumarin	8
Tincture of vanilla (10 per cent.)	50
Tincture of civet (3 per cent.)	20
Tincture of musk (3 per cent.)	20

Lavender 1218
(*after W. A. Poucher*)

	Grammes
French lavender oil	20
Bergamot oil	10
Lemon oil	2
Clary sage oil	3
Musk ambrette	1
Tincture of castoreum	5
Tincture of ambergris	25

for 1,000 alcohol.

Some Classical Recipes

Amber Lavender by Fouquet

	Grammes
Essence of lavender flowers	25
Essence of great lavender	10
Geranium oil (terpeneless)	2·5
Clove oil	1
Linalyl acetate	5
Infusion of (synthetic) ambreine	15
Infusion of musk ambrette	5
Infusion of natural civet	2·5
Infusion of benzoin	5

for 1 litre of alcohol.

Fine Amber Lavender (*Fouquet*)

	Grammes
Essence of lavender flowers	20
Great lavender oil	2·5
Clove oil	1
Sandalwood oil	0·5
Geranium oil	1·5
Linalyl acetate	5
Benzoic acid	0·5
Musk xylene	0·5
Infusion of benzoin	10
Infusion of ambrette	5
Infusion of storax	5

for 1 litre of alcohol.

Lavender Water (*Mann's Winter*)

	Grammes
Lavender oil	10
Neroli oil	0·5
Bergamot oil	10
Lemon oil	6·5
Cinnamon oil	0·5
Geranyl acetate	0·5
Isoeugenol	1·5
Coumarin	1·5
Musk ambrette	1·5
Tincture of benzoin	20
Tincture of storax	20
Tincture of tolu	20
Tincture of musk	15
Tincture of orris	60
Peru balsam	3

for 1 litre of alcohol.

Lavender Water Composition Extra (*after Cola*)

	Grammes
Lavender oil	600
Bergamot oil	100
Lemon oil	50
Geranium oil	40
Bulgarian rose oil	10
Isoeugenol	10
Coumarin	50
Musk ambrette	40
Resinodour benzoin	100

Fancy Lavender Composition (*after Cola*)

	Grammes
Lavender oil	400
Patchouli oil	10
Lemon oil	50
Citronellyl acetate	60
Geranyl acetate	100
Nerol	40
Vetiverol	20
Linalyl acetate	100
Linalyl propionate	30
Heliotropin	90
Coumarin	50
Musk ambrette	30
Musk ketone	20

Lavender-Colognes and Fancy Lavenders

It may be stressed that the linalyl acetate of lavandin can be used in place of bergamot oil, as well as of a certain proportion of lavender oil, in compositions related to oils of hesperidia (orange) and to the oils of labiatæ (lavender, rosemary, hyssop). The odour of the compositions is unchanged.

A composition for eau-de-Cologne is:

Eau-de-Cologne

	Grammes
Bergamot oil	100
Linalyl acetate	200
Lavender oil	50
Lemon oil	200
Sweet orange oil	150
Neroli oil	50
Rosemary	50
Clary sage	10
Hyssop	25
Thyme	15
Tarragon	5
Mint	5
Resinodour benzoin	100
Artificial musk and amber	40

Everyone can modify his own particular formula by following the same argument. The attempt is well worth while. One means of securing savings is to use pure lavender oil or a lavandin core not high in ester value. The outcome is usually very pleasing. Natural essences are preferable to the synthetics, since the fineness of the former is superior to that of the latter.

The term eau-de-Cologne can be applied to those products which are somewhat far removed in composition from the traditional products but are somewhat original in conception. It may well be that the name applied to the product helps its sale.

Water of Mount Caume	Grammes
Bergamot oil	100
Linalyl acetate L	250
Essence of lemon	200
Essence of Moroccan camomile	25
Essence of Portugal (sweet orange oil)	150
Rosemary	45
Clementier petitgrain oil	50
Ylang-ylang	15
Styrallyl acetate	15
Labdanum absolute	15
Soluble civet concentrate	5
Dianthax base	15
Vanillin	3
Musk ambrette	12
Resinodour benzoin	100

Lotion of Roquemartine	Grammes
Linalyl acetate L	275
Bergamot oil	165
Lemon oil	275
Portugal oil (sweet orange)	175
Rosemary	10
Petitgrain oil (bitter orange)	30
Ylang-ylang	10
Dianthax base	20
Musk ambrette	20
Panaxol base	2
Ethyl vanillin	5
Artificial amber	8
Civet	2
Indol at 100	1
Benzoin tears	2

Eau-de-Paradou	Grammes
Linalyl acetate L	390
Lemon oil	200
Geranium oil	25
Clove oil	25
Moroccan myrtle oil	25
Portugal oil (sweet orange)	40
Petitgrain oil	60
Neroli	15
Benzyl acetate	50
Resinodour benzoin	50
Resinodour tolu	25
Resinodour myrrh	25
Resinodour Peru	50
Castoreum (5 per cent.)	5
Civet (5 per cent.)	5
C_{10}-aldehyde to 10	10

Cola had given the name of a twelfth century Arabian poet to a perfume composition he had created. Some verses of the poet had inspired him: "I wept, my heart broken, sitting in the perfumed shadow of my garden."

Abou Temmam

	Grammes
Lavender oil	100
Bergamot oil	70
Rosewood oil	100
Petitgrain oil	70
Clary sage	50
Sandalwood oil	110
Geranium oil	120
Bulgarian rose oil	30
Cascarilla	60
Rock rose	30
Jasmine absolute	20
Resinodour tonka	80
Storax resinodour	90
Peru resinodour	70

It can be easily seen that the formula can be modified by different fractions of lavender oil. The manufacturers must be alive to the possibilities of the Provence essences.

Technique of Preparation

It would appear that distillation has been abandoned, since it is very much more convenient to dissolve the 100 per cent. preparation in the solvent. However, when the question is carefully weighed, it will be found that with some oils distillation is well worth while, for products of finer properties are obtained. Such losses as are incurred and such labour costs as are involved are more than amply compensated by the advantages.

Filtration cannot be avoided even when wholly soluble essences are used in the preparations. A certain number of precautions are necessary in order to obtain the crystal clearness essential in commercial products.

Both the alcoholic solution and the matured perfume acquire a certain degree of clarity as they stand. Molecular associations also take place and they alter the aroma slightly. They round off the perfume, make it homogeneous and give it the desirable properties.

Some plants incorporate a heating treatment of the perfumes to quicken the ageing. The alcoholic solutions of the essential oils are kept at 38° to 40°, over a period ranging from weeks to months, in suitable vessels connected to a central boiler. The vessels are necessarily tight and are connected through a steam trap to an adsorber containing active charcoal (carbon) to avoid losses of solvent. The method is satisfactory but expensive, and leads to a very great improvement in quality. It can be used for almost any solution, and certainly any modern plant finds such apparatus indispensable. Some firms use an oxidation process to age these solutions. They pass air or oxygen into the solutions (*cf.* the treatment of brandy), and as might be anticipated some oxidation of the terpenes will occur despite the anti-oxidant effect of the alcohol.

The solutions should be stored in well-galvanised copper containers or, better still, in stainless steel tanks, which the perfume industry regards as being much more satisfactory.

The heating process is connected to a means for cooling the product. Either the coil is directly connected with a cooling device or two circuits are installed, one for the heated liquid and the other for the cold liquid.

Attention has already been drawn to the need to guard against the apparent variation in the alcohol, due to temperature changes, and the consequent change in its solubilisation properties.

A litre of 75° alcohol, at 15°, contracts to 980·7 millilitres at 0°, but expands to 1,013 millilitres at 30°. A 75° alcohol at 15°C. has a strength of 70° G.L. at 0°C. and 79° at 30°. The essential oils will remain in solution as long as the temperature rises, but will tend to come out of solution as the temperature falls.

It is therefore essential to filter the product at the lowest temperature it is likely to reach in winter, or alternatively have a safe margin in solubility. For example, an eau-de-Cologne intended for sale at 60° should only contain sufficient oils which are soluble at 55°. The product is brought to this temperature, filtered, and the alcohol strength raised to 60° prior to being bottled. Filtration processes are almost foolproof. In bygone times fluted paper filters in smooth or fluted funnels were used, but such a method is now recognised as an uneconomic one. Hermetically closed filters are used today. One filter device consists of a filter column comprised of perforated metal discs on which suitably sized papers are placed. A central screw clamps the discs into position. Other types employ conical vessels made of phosphor bronze trellis on which a paste of filter paper or asbestos powder is placed.

Turbidity can be due to insoluble particles—*e.g.*, artificial musk—or to dust particles or to colloidal suspensions of resins or insoluble oils. When the latter is the case a substance such as magnesium carbonate, which is both wettable by the oil and can absorb it, is used. Magnesium carbonate milk or the solid itself can be mixed with the solution prior to filtration. The first runnings can be returned for further filtration if desired.

Pressure filtration is very fast. The pressure can be obtained by either placing the storage vessels at a sufficient height above the filters or by providing a source of compressed air. Plant manufacturers usually incorporate the necessary apparatus to enable the process to be easily carried out.

The operations necessary to obtain a satisfactory product have been stressed here in order to show that under present competitive conditions output in any factory, be it small or large, can only be achieved under predetermined technical control. By operating under such conditions loss of solvents is minimised and a bright clear product is obtained.

Automatic bottling and labelling machines complete the equipment.

The equipment of an unimportant small firm can be as good as that of a large concern. With present-day equipment a profitable production can be got with a very small staff. While the chemist-perfumer must be an artist, he must co-operate with an engineer. For art must be based, here as elsewhere, on science.

II. DE-LUXE EXTRACTS AND HANDKERCHIEF PERFUMES

It was pointed out, at the beginning of the second part of this work, that commercial practice has subdivided perfume products into two large groups, irrespective of the needs and wishes of customers. Merchants frequently sell lotions and eau-de-Cologne at prices which do not give them a high enough profit. They think that expensive luxury products can only be sold at a good profit, at least in certain districts. Under present economic conditions it seems that customers prefer to purchase a nice suitably sized bottle of carefully prepared perfume rather than a small bottle of more concentrated products, equally carefully prepared, at exorbitant prices.

Among lotions or toilet waters there is room for products containing 50 to 60 grammes of essential oils per litre of alcohol, as opposed to those containing 20 to 30 grammes or even 150 to 200 grammes of the absolute. Such a product would have a very wide appeal. It should be remembered that the sales technique of Americans caters for the democratisation of perfume, just as it does for cream, lipstick and powder. It is better to have all French middle-aged men and women as customers rather than a selected few.

The Formulation in Perfumery

The phenomenon of olfaction is still a mystery. Quality is entirely dependent on individual sensitivity. The manufacturer's appreciation of his own creations are only of limited value. If many customers form a similar opinion then his products are successful. On the other hand, it may be rated only a second-rate perfume—or perfumes. The value of publicity cannot be overlooked, for such publicity helps the formation of opinion. Unless a provincial creator gets some such backing his creations will never attain the success they deserve.

However, despite the fact that some formulæ have some real merits, perfumers, in general, are reluctant to try them as they are proposed, and not before they impose their own ideas on them. But what is a good perfume?

"This is," said Paul Jeancard, "a composition of different aromas whose association becomes more pleasant with time, without any false note or disharmony. There is the impression of unity which does not disturb the succession of various shades." By keeping to this definition, by following the instructions given in his manual and by using the raw materials of his stock—which are not *ipso facto* those used by the author—the manufacturer can find out for himself the probable disharmonies, the excesses, and the shortages and remedy them according to his facilities.

He will remember that Nature is still the master-perfumer. He will also recall that it is in his interest to use not only synthetic products or artificial perfumes, but essential oils in their different forms. Therefore, while use is made of synthetic perfumes obtained by analysis or synthesis, use should also be made of the natural products, the properties of which are equal, if not superior very often, to those of the synthetics.

In this way justice will keep the balance scales equal.

The formulæ given in the preceding chapters might be richer in flower oils. It is pleaded that these formulæ give relatively low priced artificial compositions and that it is useful to know how to use these compositions with greater or smaller quantities of natural oils and flower absolutes.

Bases

When reputable modern perfumes are analysed it is found that they are not made up of a large number of ingredients. On the whole they have been made with a relatively small number of materials. The original nature is to be found in some of the components used and in some unexpected notes.

In the following notes a few fashionable 100 per cent. compositions are taken and their characteristics described. When they are used in either 7 per cent. or 10 per cent. dilution they form handkerchief perfumes.

Amber 34

	Grammes
Bergamot oil	100
Jasmine absolute	15
Rose oil absolute	10
Bulgarian rose oil	10
Resinodour labdanum	40
Resinodour benzoin	80
Resinodour incense	30
Vetiver oil (terpeneless)	65
Sandalwood oil (terpeneless)	45
Rhodinol	150
Farnesol	75
Cinnamic alcohol	75
Clary sage oil	75
Heliotropin	75
Vanillin	10
Musk ketone	10
Musk ambrette	20
Ethyl vanillin	30
δ-methyl ionone	55

This composition gives an amber extract which differs but little from similar products of the last century. It will, moreover, serve as the base for many other floral compositions.

Persian Perfume 342

	Grammes
Bergamot oil	200
Jasmine oil absolute	10
Rose oil absolute	10
Bulgarian rose oil	10
Neroli oil	10
Petitgrain oil	45
Orange flower oil absolute	5
Ylang-ylang	80
Rosewood oil	45
Clary sage oil	40
Resinodour storax	10
Resinodour benzoin	50
Cinnamic alcohol	75
Benzyl acetate	20
Phenylethyl alcohol	20
Rhodinol	30
Linalyl acetate	35
Ionone and methyl ionone	150
Musk ketone	35
Musk ambrette	10
Coumarin	70
Heliotropin	40
Angelica oil	10

Here are linalyl acetate, rosewood and bergamot oils, which might have been grouped as bergamot oil. The jasmine, rose, rhodinol, cinnamic alcohol, clary sage, musks and heliotropin form a complex similar to that of the previous example. If these two groups are left out, there remain phenylethyl alcohol, rhodinol, benzyl acetate and ionone, which form an artificial rose. The petitgrain, neroli and orange flower oils form a neroli group, so that the only original notes are those due to angelica, ylang-ylang and coumarin.

The 100 per cent. Persian perfume complex could be written:

Amber compound.
Rose compound.
Neroli compound.
Ylang-ylang oil.
Angelica oil.
Coumarin.

Celesta 343

	Grammes
Bergamot oil	150
Linalool oil	35
Portugal (sweet orange) oil	35
Jasmine oil absolute	20
Benzyl acetate	35
Vetiver oil (terpeneless)	75
Sandalwood oil	35
Rhodinol or citronellol	70
Phenylethyl alcohol	100
Heliotropin	70
Vanillin	10
Musk ketone	35
Ionone	120
Neroli oil	10
Petitgrain oil (terpeneless)	50
Coumarin	80
Anisaldehyde	70

In this formula linalol and Portugal oil form a bergamot essence; benzyl acetate and neroli a jasmine. Anisaldehyde is the only original note. Thus the perfume is:

Bergamot type oil.
Synthetic amber.
Jasmine.
Neroli.
Anisaldehyde.

Care is necessary to ensure that the amber used does not contain labdanum, benzoin or clary sage.

Celesta 344

	Grammes
Bergamot oil	150
Portugal (sweet orange) oil	35
Linalol	20
Jasmine oil absolute	20
Benzyl acetate	35
Citronellol, rhodinol	70
Phenylethyl alcohol	100
Sandalwood oil	35
Neroli oil	10
Petitgrain oil	50
Heliotropin	70
Vanillin	10
Coumarin	80
Musk ketone	35
Ionone	120
Anisaldehyde	70

There is no real originality in the perfume. The first items are bergamot in type; the jasmine is benzyl acetate; the artificial rose contains neither natural absolute nor Bulgarian rose, but rhodinol, citronellol and phenylethyl alcohol. The neroli is a mixture of oils from bitter orange flowers and leaves.

This analysis leads to—

Bergamot oil,
Jasmine,
Neroli,
Rose,

with some elements of artificial amber compound.

In a similar way modern compositions could be analysed. It will be found that despite their apparent complexity the composition can be simulated by making use of alcoholic enfleurage extracts. Such recipes as the following are found:

Pomade extract of rose.
Pomade extract of jasmine.
Neroli oil.
Bergamot oil.
Tincture of amber.

Essentially this would be the perfume complex Garden 344 but diluted.

Thus it may be argued that the creation of new perfume compounds has not been of very great importance from the point of view of "harmony." But this has led to the preparation of bases, complex compositions containing the ingredients most frequently used for a certain odour, and to which may be added other notes, floral harmonies, bases and fixatives.

Use of Bases

The fact that less effort is required to make a perfume from a base has made bases more popular.

The minimum of creative spirit is necessary to use the base. A satisfactory result is obtained with the exercise of little taste, just as a designer who has an expert knowledge of colours finds little trouble in making up a coloured design. The merit of the design lies in the choice of colours. The finished product barely deserves the name of a work of art, but provided it is suitably balanced it will sell.

Better floral compositions together with the finest natural oils will improve the quality of the final product. As far as the bases themselves are concerned the trade supplies them. Alternatively they can be synthesised.

The following recipes were published in the author's earlier formulary, but because of their interest they are given again.

Carnation Base	*Grammes*
Eugenol	110
Isoeugenol	300
Acetyl isoeugenol	200
Ylang-ylang (terpeneless)	125
Rose oil, free from stearoptene	100
Santalyl acetate	50
Vanillin	50
Musk ketone	25
α-Ionone	30

Opoponax Base	*Grammes*
Bergamot oil	360
Neroli oil	20
Patchouli oil (terpeneless)	10
Bulgarian rose oil	10
Vetiverol	60
Santalol	150
Musk ambrette	40
Musk ketone	65
Castoreum absolute	40
Coumarin	80
Methyl ionone	75
Vanillin	40
Resinodour benzoin	50

Orris Base	*Grammes*
δ-Methyl ionone	660
Liquid orris	200
Concrete orris	100
Santalyl acetate	20
Vetiverol	20

Moss Base

	Grammes
Bergamot oil	125
Patchouli oil	25
Vetiverol	100
Linalol	120
Cinnamic alcohol	95
Benzyl salicylate	25
Musk ketone	100
Heliotropin	125
Coumarin	125
Artificial amber	60
Orris base (as above)	20
Resinodour Peru	50
Benzyl salicylate	25

Chypre Base

	Grammes
Bergamot oil	175
Oak moss, Evernia	50
Patchouli oil	10
Lavender oil	50
Portugal (sweet orange) oil	90
Sandalwood oil	50
Crystalline cedrol	80
Geraniol, palmarosa	110
Safrol	10
Coumarin	50
Musk ambrette	25
Musk ketone	50
Heliotropin	100
Ionone	60
Artificial jasmine	40
Resinodour Peru	50

Wood Base

	Grammes
Bergamot oil	250
Bulgarian rose oil	50
Sandalwood oil (terpeneless)	40
Vetiver oil (terpeneless)	110
Crystalline cedrol	50
Cinnamyl acetate	40
Cinnamic alcohol	80
Coumarin	70
Methyl ionone	150
Resinodour Peru	40
Benzyl acetate	60
Musk ketone	40
Musk ambrette	20

These bases are balanced formulations—*i.e.*, they contain the correct balance of main, floral and fixing ingredients. Whatever the amount of base used, there is no risk whatsoever of producing a product which lacks balance.

In some cases the bases can be diluted in alcohol, but it is desirable to add other ingredients in order to give the product some originality.

The following examples are quite well known:

Orichalque 7

		Grammes
Main odour:	Bergamot oil	120
Floral:	Jasmin complex	75
	Liquid orris	30
	Rose complex	80
Base:	Opoponax	665
	Vetiver oil	25
Fixative:	Civettone	5

A different bouquet will result if other roses are chosen—*e.g.*, red, moss, calyx, etc. Similarly, the quality of the jasmine will strongly affect the final composition's aroma.

If the model formula is simplified variations can be worked out.

By using a mixture of tangerine, lemon and orange oils in place of bergamot oil a completely different extract will result.

Saphir 19

		Grammes
Main bouquet:	Bergamot oil	100
Floral:	Fern composition	150
	Bouvardia composition ..	100
	Jasmine composition ..	75
Base:	Opoponax	475
	Santalol	20
	Coumarin	40
Fixative:	Tincture of musk ketone ..	40

Spring Air 27

		Grammes
Main bouquet:	Essence of aurantiacæ ..	25
Floral:	Artificial lilac extra ..	125
	Rose compound	30
Base:	Wood base	700
	Vetiverol	100
Fixative:	Musk ketone	20

Sky Blue 162

Without main:

		Grammes
Floral:	Jasmine compound ..	225
	Orris compound	200
	Rose compound	110
Base:	Wood base	125
	Vetiverol or cedrol ..	95
Fixative:	Musk ketone	50

These formulæ reflect the 1935 ideas; those of recent years have new notes.

Perfumers then introduced characteristic new shades of bouquets. They used and abused the aldehyde odour and later introduced the composition known as Russian leather, particularly for men's toiletries.

Lastly, with the rise in demand for exclusively masculine odours, search was made for such bouquets as tobacco, island wood, and improved variations of the preceding formulæ.

Indications on the preparation of such bouquets will be given later.

Perfumes for Men

The main concern of perfumers has been to win female customers. They have succeeded.

Male customers are much more reserved. Why should men use perfumes? History tells us that men did use them and that they sometimes used them to excess. Can it be said that the modern man resists the lure of healthy, clean and quiet perfumes? Must the business man surround himself in tobacco, the odour of which is disliked in some quarters? And must petrol, benzene and oil with their smells be the sole right of some men?

This is a matter of suitably worded advertisements. Some discerning sellers concentrate on such an approach and then, having interested the male element who are interested in art and fashion, find that the mass follows.

The endeavour is to create some summation of odours that will inspire and be reminders of activity and freedom and sports. The most recommended are those of chypre, lavender, tobacco and wood, and these will be discussed in the present chapter.

Chypres

The odoriferous balsams of the Chypre island held undisputed sway for thousands of years. Ancient pottery of the Bronze Age was found to have contained, or so it appears, essences or oils which were rich in resinous balsams. (The pottery is found on the whole Mediterranean coast.) Rose and labdanum, among other local plants, must have had a part in them.

The modern chypres have preserved something of their ancient make-up, for they use resinous wood, amber rock rose, oak moss and other flowers.

The well-known chypre of Coty brought this note back into fashion, and there it has remained for the last twenty-five years. Everybody sought to have his own chypre. Some have used rustic notes such as that of artemisia and very feminine essences such as clary sage, or even the lively pleasing notes of nutmeg oil. Other makers have introduced the spicy note particularly for men.

The following examples illustrate some of the many variations of the chypre theme:

CHYPRE COMPOSITIONS

Chypre I

	Grammes
Linalol of rosewood	100
Linalol of lavandin	100
Bergamot oil	200
Wood complex	150
Dianthax base	80
Methyl ionone	90
Pimento oil	95
Petitgrain oil	80
Portugal guinea oil	40
Essence of spices No. 1	10
Oak moss absolute	40
Coumarin	60
Heliotropin	75
Musk xylene	40

Chypre II

	Grammes
Wood complex	100
Terpineol	100
Phenylethyl alcohol	100
Resinodour benzoin	90
Linalol	60
Benzyl acetate	90
Patchouli oil	20
Isoeugenol	55
Artemisia oil (Moroccan)	40
Geraniol	90
Ionone	45
Oak moss absolute	5
Isobutyl salicylate	20
Coumarin	50
Heliotropin	100
Resinodour tonka	35

Chypre III

	Grammes
Linalol of lavandin	330
Linalyl acetate of lavender	110
Amyl salicylate	100
Wood complex	60
Isoeugenol	20
Safrol	10
Benzyl acetate	35
Ionone	30
Coumarin	60
Ethyl vanillin	35
Heliotropin	90
Musk ambrette	25

Chypre IV

	Grammes
Bergamot oil	260
Clary sage oil	50
Lavender oil	30
Tarragon oil	15
Oil of hyssop	10
Rosewood oil	50
Neroli	10
French rose oil	5
Wood complex	175
Labdanum absolute	55
Oak moss absolute	30
Jasmine absolute	25
Isoeugenol	20
Methyl ionone	100
Coumarin	75
Heliotropin	40
Musk ketone	50

Chypre V

	Grammes
Bergamot oil	160
Portugal oil	30
Complex of wood essences	130
Terpineol	120
Lavender oil	20
Geraniol	110
Ionone	55
Benzyl acetate	40
Peru balsam	30
Coumarin	45
Heliotropin	100
Cassia absolute	10
Oak moss absolute	30
Labdanum absolute	45
Musk xylene	55
Musk ambrette	15

Chypre Super VI

	Grammes
Sandalwood oil	50
Tarragon oil	25
Angelica root oil	5
Clary sage oil	30
Vetiver oil	60
Lavandin	50
Patchouli oil	20
Bergamot oil	225
Ylang-ylang	95
Oak moss	60
Coumarin	90
Labdanum resinodour	25
Isoeugenol	35
Methyl ionone	50
Jasmine absolute	10
Orris extra	15
Cinnamyl acetate	25
Vanillin	20
Heliotropin	20
Musk ambrette	20
Musk ketone	30
Resinodour benzoin	50

Chypre (English Taste) VII

	Grammes
Bergamot oil	440
Petitgrain oil (Tunisian)	85
Sandalwood oil	80
Patchouli oil	5
Lemon oil (terpeneless)	10
Cedar oil	10
Artificial rose	85
Artificial jasmine	80
Methyl ionone	80
Isoeugenol	40
Vanillin	40
Coumarin	15
Labdanum absolute	15
Artificial musk	15

Chypre VIII

	Grammes
Bergamot oil	225
Vetiver oil	75
Patchouli oil	10
Sandalwood oil	70
Ylang-ylang	65
Oak moss	50
Isoeugenol	35
Benzyl acetate	50
Rhodinol	80
Benzyl salicylate	70
Cinnamic alcohol	50
Coumarin	70
Heliotropin	100
Musk ketone	50

Leather Perfumes

The leather perfumes like those of chypre were created to please the male customers. Alfred de Musset was delighted with the odour of Russian leather. Villiers de l'Isle Adam spread news of it in his way. Spanish leather perfumes, rich in civet, no longer have an appeal. On the other hand, more recent creations have become popular and remain so.

Still, much remains to be done. If it is possible there should be an element of the animal in the perfume, yet the whole perfume should be clean and fresh. It should appeal to the discerning man.

Russian Leather

	Grammes
Pyrogenous essence of cedar, Portion II	50
Wood complex	125
Clary sage oil	50
Bergamot oil	50
Cinnamic alcohol	100
Geranyl acetate	70
Benzyl acetate	50
Isoeugenol	50
Eugenol	50
Terpineol	25
Geraniol	75
Citronellol	40
Ethyl vanillin	45
Artificial amber	60
Resinodour labdanum	130
Musk ambrette	40
Concentrated castoreum	10
Concentrated civet	15

Leather Base

	Grammes
Anisyl acetate	20
Ethyl anisate	40
Rectified pyrogenous cedar I	50
Methyl salicylate	10
Storax	150
Peru balsam	150
Ethyl vanillin	20
Artificial amber	50
Terpineol	280
Benzyl benzoate	230

Tobacco Flowers

At the moment, although many manufacturers toy with the idea, there is no question of finding odours which are complementary to those left after the pipe has been used, the cigar and cigarette smoked. Men and women smokers are appreciative of perfumes which arouse in them memories of the smell of some particularly scented tobacco. These perfumes do not have the bouquet of oriental tobacco, or of Havanas, or of certain American cigarettes, but they do correct the unbearable stale odours of these products smoked indoors.

Varieties of Solanaceæ, with their bouquet of tobacco, are distilled or extracted with solvents, and the products sold under the name of Tabacine I, II, etc.

	Grammes
Artificial tobacco M	350
Natural absolute of tabacine	50
Artificial jasmine	50
Methyl ionone	60
Labdanum absolute	60
Cassia absolute	20
Artificial cassia	20
Tuberose absolute	10
Heliotropin	70
Vanillin	10
Vetiverol	60
Neroli oil	30
Rose oil	40
Orange flower oil	20
Coumarin	50
Aroma of beeswax	40
Russian leather complex	20
Musk ketone	40

Tobacco Flavours

The sale of perfume compositions for flavouring cigarettes, cigars and pipe tobacco is very restricted in France as there are very few flavoured products.

These compositions are, however, sold for export. It will therefore be of some advantage to have a knowledge of their make-up, particularly as such knowledge helps in catering for the tastes of men. By combining together either the aroma of tobacco flowers or that of wood complexes with the bouquet of English, American or Oriental cigarettes, some good effects are obtained.

Flavour for Cigar-box

	Grammes
American cedar oil	500
Vetiver oil	20
Chinese cinnamon oil	2
Tabacine II	20
Clove oil	8
Crystalline cedrol	200
Hydroxycitronellal	250

Sumatra Flower

	Grammes
Cedarwood oil	500
Lavender oil	50
Amboine clove oil	50
Calamus oil	30
Methyl isoeugenol	25
Coumarin	200
Eugenol	50
Resinodour labdanum	90
C_{16}-aldehyde	10
Amber fixative	235

London Perfume

	Grammes
Orange oil (Guinea)	300
Cinnamon oil	40
Cascarilla oil	100
Mace-nutmeg oil	160
Clove oil	60
Rose oil	60
Coumarin	100
Heliotropin	40
Vanillin	40
Resinodour tonka	100

Camel-type Flavour

	Grammes
Lavender oil	150
Cinnamon oil	330
Cardamom oil	30
Celery	25
Artificial honey essence	25
Vanillin	150
Undecalactone	25

Virginia Flavour

	Grammes
Bergamot oil	120
Orange oil	80
Lemon oil	110
Cinnamon oil	20
Geranium oil	200
Clove oil	60
Ethyl vanillin	65
Methyl ionone	65
Ethyl valerianate	5
Resinodour tonka	275

Virginia II

	Grammes
Geranium oil	400
Lavender oil	100
Bergamot oil	60
Clove oil	10
Rose oil	20
Orange oil (Guinea)	100
Cascarilla oil	30
Methyl ionone	60
Coumarin	70
Vanillin	30
Ethyl valerianate	5
Resinodour tonka	125

Clay

	Grammes
Sassafras oil	380
Ceylon cinnamon oil	80
Indo-China cedar oil	50
Heliotropin	130
Methyl isoeugenol	150
Resinodour mastic	30
Resinodour storax	180

"Three Castle" Flavour

	Grammes
Essence of ginger	135
Clove oil	60
Cardamom oil	35
Chinese cinnamon oil	255
Isoeugenol	90
Vanillin	220
Butyl butyrate	10

Brazil Flavour

	Grammes
Bergamot oil	400
Cinnamon oil	200
Cascarilla oil	180
Bitter almond oil	10
Butyl butyrate	10
Resinodour storax	200

Player's Flavour

	Grammes
Bergamot oil	300
Cinnamon oil	290
Cardamom oil	25
Caraway oil	5
Clove oil	175
Ethyl butyrate	5
Resinodour vanilla	100

"Lucky" Perfume Type

	Grammes
Cinnamon oil	500
Clove oil	250
Lavender oil	150
Oil of fennel	25
Vanillin	50
Benzyl butyrate	25

"Kentucky" Flavour

	Grammes
Cinnamon oil	600
Oil of fennel	150
Lavender oil	100
Undecalactone	50
Ethyl valerianate	50
Ethyl butyrate	50

"Havana" Flavour

	Grammes
Cedar oil	350
Tabacine II	20
Resinodour storax	250
Resinodour labdanum	50
Methyl isoeugenol	300
Resinodour mastic	30

"Havana" II

	Grammes
Clove oil	300
Cascarilla oil	200
Rose oil	50
Tabacine oil	100
Cedar oil	100
Vanillin	100
Coumarin	150

"Manila" Flavour

	Grammes
Chinese cinnamon oil	100
Cascarilla oil	75
Benzyl isoeugenol	250
Coumarin	150
Vanillin	120
Ethyl butyrate	5
Resinodour storax	300

"Manila II"

	Grammes
Cedar oil	500
Geranium oil	250
Patchouli oil	50
Sandalwood oil	200

"Alexandria" Flavour

	Grammes
Artificial jasmine	75
Artificial rose	30
Coumarin	75
Musk ketone	75
Heliotropin	75
Resinodour olibanum	75
Resinodour labdanum	600

Oriental Tobacco

	Grammes
Artificial jasmine	350
Artificial orange flower	50
Cinnamon oil	100
Artificial rose	100
Vanillin	100
Resinodour tonka	300

Perfume "Ankara" I

	Grammes
Tobacco flower M	475
Phorax base	100
Phenylethyl acetate	20
Coumarin	80
Cinnamic alcohol	70
Heliotropin	60
Artificial amber	50
Artificial rose	20
Artificial jasmine	30
Linalyl acetate	90
C_{12}-aldehyde	5

"Ankara" II

	Grammes
Geranium oil	180
Neroli oil	100
Rose oil	100
Tuberose	60
Jasmine oil	40
Lavender oil	160
Patchouli oil	40
Celery oil	40
Vanillin	15
Methyl ionone	140
Ethyl phenacetate	20
Resinodour tonka	115

Wood Perfumes

Wood perfumes are reminiscent of the pleasing sensation experienced when cedarwood pencils were used, sometimes by scholars, sometimes by bookkeepers who loved to bite and chew chips. The discovery of some methyl ionones with an odour of cedar has lent importance to the introduction of woody notes into luxury perfumes. But there has been insufficient study of the complexes which can simulate the odour of the luxurious "Island wood" box, or that of the African or Polynesian wooden carved charm, or even that of the indefinable subtle yet effective bouquets of some furniture.

There is ample room for progress in this field.

Wood Compositions

Most modern perfumes contain some proportion of wood essences. The essences contribute to the persistence of the perfumes and, with crystalline odoriferous materials of low vapour pressure, form blended bases.

It is, of course, desirable to know that compounders display a lack of originality and limit themselves to the use of the same three or four essences, those of sandalwood, vetiver, cedar and patchouli, together with the esters of santalol, vetiverol and cedrol. Some useful variations result when these ingredients are substituted by derivatives from the same sylvestrian series. American perfumers largely employ cedrol and its acetate, both of which have a delicate "pencilwood" odour almost as pleasant as that of orris. The Virginian cedar oils are usually rich in an almost insoluble sesquiterpene and contain but traces of cedrol. It appears as though French perfumers will have to await the resumption of distillation in Indo-China for really suitable sources.

Cedrenol and Peu-Mousol are very like sandalwood oil and they can be suitably modified by some synthetics. Crude cypress oil sometimes replaces lemon oil and introduces an original note. The terpeneless product has a fine amber perfume.

The first example illustrates a modern formula. It contains larger quantities of wood essences than do the others.

Indian Wood 8

	Grammes
Essence of sandalwood	115
Crystalline cedrol	75
δ-Methyl ionone	75
Cypress oil	38
Ylang-ylang	25
Geranium oil	25
Patchouli oil	15
Vetiver oil	75
Artificial rose	300
Geranyl acetate	25
Artificial amber	30
Ethyl vanillin	12
Coumarin	25
Musk ambrette	30
Musk xylene	25

The following yields a real wood odour and it can also be used as a starting point for men's perfume.

Pagodes

	Grammes
Sandalwood oil	150
Methyl ionone	100
Cedrol	35
Vetiveryl acetate	35
Essence of bergamot	170
Civet absolute	50
Caraway oil	20
Rosewood oil	75
Real rose oil	5
Lavender oil	50
Coumarin	95
Vanillin	5
Resinodour opoponax	75

Gilded Wood

	Grammes
Methyl ionone	200
Ionone	200
Cedryl acetate	100
Cinnamic alcohol	100
Heliotropin	100
Neroli oil	20
Petitgrain oil	20
Ylang-ylang	40
Benzyl acetate	80
Essence of Rhodes wood	40
Musk ambrette	50
Musk ketone	50

Siam Wood

	Grammes
Rectified oil of Peu Mou	90
Vetiver oil	60
Cedryl acetate	100
Methyl ionone	225
Cedrenol	50
Guaiacum wood oil	25
Amyl phenylacetate	60
Citronellyl formate	80
Bergamot oil	150
Artificial rose	25
Jasmine absolute	20
Coumarin	80

Palissander

	Grammes
δ-Methyl ionone	150
β-Ionone	80
Orris resinoid	80
Peu-moussol	200
Anisaldehyde	40
Vetiver oil	90
Neroli oil	50
Bergamot oil	50
Dacridium oil	100
Rosewood oil	30
Benzyl acetate	80
Musk xylene	50

Havana Wood

	Grammes
Wood essences, complex	250
Ionone	250
Ylang-ylang	15
Bergamot oil	55
Geraniol	50
Resinodour tolu	30
Resinodour labdanum	50
Resinodour incense	50
Concentrated castoreum	20
Heliotropin	70
Musk ambrette	70
Musk ketone	60
Musk xylene	30

Angelwood (Aldehydes)

	Grammes
Dacridium oil	180
Vetiver oil	65
Methyl ionone	90
Leather base (see above)	30
Artificial rose	75
Artificial jasmine	90
Dianthax	80
Resinoid of labdanum	40
Oak moss absolute	20
Cinnamic alcohol	100
Heliotropin	40
Musk ambrette	40
Coumarin	55
Vanillin	25
Musk xylene	40
C_8-C_{10}-aldehyde	10
C_9-C_{10}-aldehyde	10
C_{10}-aldehyde	10

Floral Fancies

It cannot be too well known that although chemistry provided perfumers with new products, the perfumers limited their outlook to bouquets based on old ideas. They prepared artificial flower oils and used them in much the same way as natural oils. It will be said that benzyl acetate does not simulate the jasmine bouquet, but that it is an ingredient contributing to it; further, that amyl salicylate or isobutyl phenacetate really imparts new notes to the composition, and finally that vanillin, heliotropin and synthetic musks have really warranted the preparation of clinging, persistent bouquets.

This, however, is no longer correct, and yet modern perfumery pursues its way.

Apart from such improvements, the majority of modern compositions are variations upon modified classical floral themes improved with new notes, both natural and synthetic. While this is not unimportant, it proves that Nature has so far provided us with such perfect models of an unsurpassed quality that nothing better is possible than to imitate her, and that the summations of all efforts to create something new are the more or less original, and more or less successful bouquets. The long involved formulæ, of which manufacturers are so proud, lose their complexity when they are broken up into their real components and the synthetic products are grouped under the name of the flowers the odour of which they help to simulate. Variations on lilac, rose violet and amber perfumes will be studied. It is essential that these bouquets should be accompanied by the so-called "head" odours, the lighter and more volatile ones—to accord with the olfactory mechanism—as well as by heavier and less volatile bouquets, the bases or fixatives. Cedrat bouquets and those of complexes similar to those used to prepare eau-de-Cologne are examples of the lighter odours.

The bouquets of white flowers such as orange-flower, jasmine, bouvardia, hawthorn, narcissus, or those of red flowers or roses, purple lilac, cyclamen, rose, and leaves, can be thought of in this way. Other perfumes will be complexes with the bouquet of wood or leather or chypre, and now the cycle of Nature's gifts is complete.

The compounder's part is restricted to the purchase of the best synthetic floral compositions or, provided he has the means, to their preparation. His opportunities to do so are so rare, for creative artists do not readily release their characteristic novelties as they seek to create inimitable specialties. If he can marry, as the young Japanese do, form and floral colours in symphonies, he will create tasteful innovations, generally summarised in ten-line formulæ. These ten lines will have as much value as those of fifty or more put forward by compounders who add yet another stone to their unfinished building. Builders of the golden age used majestic, evenly squared or carved stones and laid them in well-balanced foundations. Modern builders reduce the stone to dust and powder and with them make cement with which they erect buildings. Perfumers are doing the same.

Lilac

Lilac perfume was not available earlier to the perfumer. The introduction of hydroxycitronellal, together with the combinations of this ingredient with new elements, has facilitated the reconstitution of a lilac bouquet of such perfection that it has been used in a hundred different ways. For twenty years perfumery has been dominated by lilac. But the fashion of today likes whims, so the most outstanding lilacs are sold under a fanciful name rather than under its true name. Care has been taken by the author to avoid imitating compositions which are fashionable. As the inspiration of the professional sometimes depends on reminiscences, an apology is offered to those creative artists who may be unable to recognise their masterpieces.

While nitrated musks are mentioned in some recipes, they are not included readily.

Lilac I

	Grammes
Best artificial lilac	800
"Complex" essence of ylang-ylang	40
Jasmine absolute	10
α-Ionone	90
Musk ketone	20
Musk ambrette	40

Lilac II

	Grammes
Artificial lilac	550
Hydroxycitronellal	100
Ylang-ylang (first grade)	50
Jasmine absolute	50
Rose absolute	25
α-Ionone	25
Phenylethyl alcohol	50
Heliotropin	50
Musk ketone	50

Lilac III

	Grammes
Artificial lilac	560
Artificial lily of the valley	140
Ylang-ylang (first grade)	60
Hydroxycitronellal	40
Moroccan rose absolute	20
Jasmine absolute	50
Civet absolute	10
Heliotropin	80
Musk ketone	50

Lilac IV

	Grammes
Artificial lilac (extra)	560
Ylang-ylang (complete)	100
Bulgarian or French rose	20
Cinnamic alcohol	60
Heliotropin	70
Musk ketone	20
Musk ambrette	20

Lilac V

	Grammes
Lilac extra	400
Ylang-ylang (first grade)	100
Cinnamic alcohol	100
Phenylacetic aldehyde (10 per cent.)	25
Benzyl acetate	25
Hydroxycitronellal	25
α-Amyl cinnamic aldehyde	25
Linalyl acetate	50
Jasmine absolute	10
Jasmine "frame"	45
Rose absolute	10
Heliotropin	80
Musk ketone	50

Lilac Variation—First

	Grammes
Artificial lilac (extra)	250
Ylang-ylang (first grade)	250
Phorax base	250
Artificial jasmine	150
Heliotropin	150
Musk ketone	20
Musk ambrette	50

Second Variation

	Grammes
Artificial lilac (extra)	130
Lily of the valley (extra)	100
Ylang-ylang (first grade)	100
Jasmine absolute	15
Rose absolute	20
French rose oil	10
Linalol of rosewood	20
Panaxol base	35
Wood complex	20
Artificial rose	100
Methyl ionone	55
Eau-de-Cologne essence	80
Tarragon oil	20
Angelica oil	30
Resinaroma benzoin	50
Resinaroma incense	20
Heliotropin	60
Musk ambrette	35
Musk ketone	30

Third Variation

	Grammes
Artificial lilac (extra)	360
Jasmine "frame"	60
Jasmine absolute	30
Ylang-ylang (first grade)	10
Clary sage oil	25
Angelica oil	45
α-Ionone	75
Methyl ionone	65
Orange flower absolute	20
Cassia absolute	20
Rose absolute	30
Anisaldehyde	15
Wood complex	50
Heliotropin	90
Coumarin	80
Musk ketone	35
Musk ambrette	5

Fourth Variation

	Grammes
Artificial lilac (extra)	225
Jasmine absolute	15
Rose absolute	20
French rose	20
Methyl ionone	100
Phorax or sophora base	150
Resinodour incense	25
Resinodour tolu	25
Resinodour benzoin	50
Wood complex	125
Ambreine labdanum	5
Artificial amber	60
Musk ketone	25
Musk ambrette	20

Fifth Variation

	Grammes
Artificial lilac (extra)	225
Ylang-ylang (first grade)	235
Artificial jasmine (extra)	100
Artificial lily of the valley (extra)	180
Artificial rose (extra)	60
Tuberose absolute	50
Methylnonyl acetic aldehyde (10 per cent.)	20
Heliotropin	60
Musk ketone	30

Sixth Variation

	Grammes
Artificial lilac (extra)	500
Artificial lily of the valley (extra)	100
Ylang-ylang (first grade)	100
Jasmine " frame "	50
Ionone	35
Bulgarian rose	25
C_{12}-aldehyde (10 per cent.)	25
Heliotropin	75
Musk ketone	50

Seventh Variation

	Grammes
Artificial lilac (extra)	250
Artificial lily of the valley	220
Ylang-ylang	35
Artificial rose	82
Jasmine absolute	6·5
Cedrat oil	85
Amyl salicylate	88
Wood complex	20
Labdanum absolute	35
Orange absolute	1
Orris absolute (10 per cent.)	15
Resinodour storax	15
Artificial amber	3·5
Civet absolute	1
C_{10}-aldehyde (50 per cent.)	20
Methyl nonyl acetaldehyde (1 per cent.)	14
Ethyl vanillin	3
Musk ketone	35
Musk ambrette	70
Heliotropin	1

Eighth Variation

	Grammes
Artificial lilac (extra)	360
Artificial jasmine	180
Ylang-ylang (first grade)	70
Benzyl salicylate	50
Rose absolute	10
Labdanum absolute	70
Panaxol base	60
Bergamot oil	70
Vanillin	10
Coumarin	25
Heliotropin	50
Musk ketone	25
Musk ambrette	30

Ninth Variation

	Grammes
Artificial lilac (extra)	700
Artificial jasmine	40
Jasmine absolute	10
Ylang-ylang (first grade)	20
Benzyl salicylate	30
Hydroxycitronellal	60
C_{10}-C_{12}-aldehyde	10
Vanillin	10
Heliotropin	40
Musk ketone	60

Rose

The rose is not in fashion because it, like the world, is very old. But it will come again. It is to be found throughout the whole world and is an ingredient of most, if not all, perfumes. Apparently no perfume can claim perfection without it.

Some years ago the rose was the foundation for the fortune of a very famous perfumer. His creation was a luxurious product, yet in very good taste.

Rose I

	Grammes
Artificial rose (extra)	650
Rose absolute	100
Bulgarian rose oil	100
Ionone	150
Methyl ionone	40
Jasmine absolute	10
Musk ketone	50

Rose II

	Grammes
Bulgarian rose oil	200
Rose absolute	200
Rhodinol	200
Guaiacol acetate	50
Methyl ionone	50
Rhodinyl acetate	50
Santalyl acetate	50
Phenylethyl alcohol	60
Phenylacetic acid	10
Terpeneless palmarosa	110
Musk ketone	20

Rose Variation—First

	Grammes
Rose compound	695
Artificial lily of the valley	150
Methyl ionone	65
Jasmine compound	15
Heliotropin	25
Musk ketone	50

By the term "rose compound" is understood a mixture of artificial and natural essences in contradistinction to the artificial product, which consists of synthetics. Jasmine compound is a mixture of natural and artificial essences.

Second Variation

	Grammes
Artificial rose	260
Cologne composition	400
Artificial carnation	30
Nutmeg oil	20
Wood complex	80
Jasmine compound	60
Tuberose absolute	15
Vanillin	45
Heliotropin	10
Coumarin	40
Musk ambrette	35
Musk ketone	5

Variation—Lily, Lily of the Valley, Rose and Narcissus

	Grammes
Oriental rose composition	160
Artificial lily of the valley (extra)	340
Artificial lilac (extra)	200
Cinnamic alcohol	100
Artificial narcissus	65
Phenylacetic aldehyde	10
Heliotropin	75
Musk ketone	50

Violet and Iris

The discovery of ionone and then of methyl ionone with odours intermediate between that of iris (orris) and that of cedarwood has powerfully influenced not only violet perfumes but others. It can be said that methyl ionone only has a violet odour when fully diluted. The compounds, however, contribute their share to rose perfumes, as will be seen in the last chapter. It thus takes its place in many compositions. Under certain conditions the methyl ionones are reminders of iris and they blend well with wood complexes, and in addition play an undefined but pleasant rôle in many mixtures.

It will be seen how easy it is to use these materials.

In violet bouquets both natural and synthetic (methyl heptine carbonate) leaf fragrances are used, since the public does not distinguish between the fragrances of the leaf and flower.

Violet

	Grammes
α-Ionone	600
Methyl ionone	30
Absolute of violet flowers	30
Absolute of violet leaves	10
Benzyl acetate	20
Concrete orris	50
Ylang-ylang	30
Jasmine compound	110
Parma violet complex	40
Heliotropin	80

Violet Variation—First

	Grammes
Ionone	125
Methyl ionone	75
Linalol	100
Phenylethyl alcohol	75
Cinnamic alcohol	125
Terpineol	50
Benzyl acetate	40
Cologne complex	200
Amyl salicylate	25
Isoeugenol	40
Heliotropin	100
Musk ambrette	50

Second Variation

	Grammes
Methyl ionone	400
Wood complex	50
Neroli oil	75
Bergamot oil	20
Isoeugenol	150
Benzyl acetate	50
Rose compound	25
Coumarin	150
Musk ketone	50
Musk ambrette	30

Third Variation

	Grammes
Methyl ionone	350
Ionone	80
Cassia absolute	70
Jasmine compound	95
Concrete orris	35
Lilac (extra)	180
Rose compound	30
Bergamot oil	60
Vanillin	20
Heliotropin	40
Coumarin	40

AMBER

The odour of amber, as imagined by the public, bears little relation to that of true, unsuspected, even unknown tincture of amber. It has a hot, strong, powerful smell which is increased by the addition of animal perfumes, musk, civet and castoreum (male parasexual secretions) and given perhaps a feminine touch by clary sage oil.

Thus amber perfume could be classified along with those of leather, tobacco, lavender and chypre as essentially masculine in appeal, and might appeal to a large circle who do not usually use perfumes.

In the past soldiers could recall the smell of their mounts (horse—metacresyl phenylacetate) or that of their harness (Russian leather). What can they recall today? Nothing but the smell of dirty oil. So why should they not in some way recompense themselves? Civilians having acquired the habit of using perfumes, can find many occasions on which to do so.

Amber compounds contain, as has already been mentioned, the previously mentioned animal perfumes. The synthetic substitutes, as well as labdanum and oak moss absolutes, contain such spice oils as nutmeg, mace, opoponax, ambrette and certain balsams, as well as spicy seeds.

Amber blends readily with Spanish skin. (This was originally a skin impregnated with civet and wood perfumes enriched with amber.)

Amber, popular as it is, is often used to impart tenacious and heady properties to floral novelties. This is the explanation for limiting the examples which follow and which could be readily combined with earlier ones.

Amber

	Grammes
Labdanum absolute	75
Tincture of ambergris	150
Musk ambrette	75
Absolute of oak moss	25
Vetiver oil	75
Rose absolute	25
α-Ionone	150
Vanillin	50
Heliotropin	70
Resinaroma benzoin	115
Cinnamic alcohol	190

Amber Variation—First

	Grammes
Labdanum absolute	45
Liquid artificial amber	175
Tincture of ambergris	25
Clary sage oil	25
Musk ketone	60
Musk ambrette	60
Benzoin 50 per cent. resinaroma	225
Methyl ionone	75
Wood complex	80
Artificial rose	155
Jasmine absolute	10
Heliotropin	50
Vanillin	15

Second Variation

	Grammes
Liquid artificial amber	300
Bergamot oil	200
Rose oil absolute	50
Resinodour tolu	150
Ionone	240
Musk ketone	40
Musk ambrette	20

Third Variation Analysed

	Grammes
Amber:	
Vanillin	80
Coumarin	65
Heliotropin	20
Amber in pieces	24
Clary sage	15
Musk xylene	80
Civet absolute	3
Resinodour benzoin	75
Resinodour storax	10
Resinodour labdanum	8
Resinodour vanilla	50
Coriander oil	80
Wood complex:	
Sandalwood oil	100
Vetiver oil	50
Patchouli oil	30
Floral:	
Jasmine absolute	15
Rose absolute	10
Concrete orris	30
Methyl ionone	5
Lavender absolute	15
"Head" odour:	
Lemon oil	50
Neroli oil	5
Bergamot oil	150

FANCY ODOURS FREE OF DOMINANT NOTES

Most modern perfumes are bouquets in which a particularly successful modified note cannot be distinguished. They are bouquets in the truest sense of the word, for the fragrances of dissimilar flowers are blended with great artistry. A modern perfume, in which lily of the valley is blended with orange flower as the "head" notes, together with balsam and aldehyde notes, can be made to the following:

Modern Perfume

	Grammes
Orange oil (Guinea)	215
Bergamot oil	150
Neroli oil (Bigarade)	15
Ylang-ylang (Bourbon)	65
Jasmine oil absolute	15
Orange flower oil absolute	15
Rose oil absolute	15
Clary sage oil	15
Artificial lily of the valley (extra)	150
Panaxol base	90
Artificial jasmine (extra)	75
Methyl nonyl acetaldehyde (5 per cent.)	15
C_9-aldehyde (5 per cent.)	30
Heliotropin	75
Vanillin	30
Musk xylene	30

100 grammes to be dissolved in 1 litre of alcohol. 25 grammes of a 3 per cent. tincture of natural musk to be added, as well as 25 grammes of amber or other natural fixative.

The following is a more economical, simplified version of the foregoing formula.

Simplified Modern Perfume

	Grammes
Vetiver oil	50
Bergamot oil	50
Jasmine oil absolute	10
Rose oil absolute	10
Neroli oil	10
Sweet orange oil (Guinea)	60
Nerol	280
Cinnamic alcohol	100
Panaxol base	200
Benzyl acetate	40
Methyl ionone	75
Methyl nonyl acetaldehyde (10 per cent.)	50
C_9-aldehyde (10 per cent.)	20
Musk xylene	50

The formulæ are said to be developed when the constituents of the complexes are given—*e.g.*, those of artificial jasmine, artificial lily of the valley, artificial rose. Frequently they contain commercial synthetics either because the nature of such products is unknown or because their fragrance cannot be simulated. Most recipes are mixtures. The longest formulæ are not always the best, but such is the vanity of some manufacturers that they make their formulæ longer than those of their competitors.

Malta

	Grammes
Tangerine oil	60
Lemon oil	175
Vetiver oil	15
Ylang-ylang	60
Cedrol	60
Artificial tuberose	100
Ionone	100
Phenylethyl alcohol	160
Cinnamic alcohol	50
C_{10}-aldehyde	25
Methyl nonyl acetaldehyde	20
Ethyl vanillin	30
Heliotropin	50
Resinodour benzoin	50
Musk ketone	50

Mutellina

	Grammes
Bergamot oil	260
Vetiver oil	150
Oak moss	40
Hydroxycitronellal	90
Geranyl acetate	90
Styrallyl acetate	10
Rhodinol	25
Geraniol	90
Phenylacetic aldehyde	30
Cinnamic alcohol	90
Vanillin	45
Heliotropin	50
Musk ambrette	30

Meryanthe

	Grammes
Bergamot oil	75
Jasmine oil absolute	25
Clove oil	100
Tarragon oil	25
Labdanum oil absolute	50
Benzyl acetate	50
Phenylethyl alcohol	50
Cinnamic alcohol	175
Phorax base	225
Cinnamic aldehyde	25
Vanillin	100
Musk ketone	50
Musk ambrette	50

Satin Bouquet

	Grammes
Oak moss	160
Sandalwood oil	40
Ylang-ylang	35
Bulgarian rose oil	20
Rose oil absolute	10
Patchouli oil	10
Costus oil	5
Artificial jasmine (extra)	160
Methyl ionone	100
Cinnamic alcohol	35
Phenylethyl alcohol	35
Vetiveryl acetate	35
Styrallyl acetate	10
Hydroxycitronellal	35
Linalol	35
Dianthax base	10
Cinnamic aldehyde	10
Dimethylhydrocinnamol	20
Artificial gardenia	100
Vanillin	10
C_{10}-aldehyde	5
C_{11}-aldehyde	25
Musk ambrette	10
Musk ketone	20

Kafka

	Grammes
Bergamot oil	225
Clary sage oil	2
Oil of rue	1
Ylang-ylang	50
Petitgrain oil	40
Ionone	100
Geraniol	165
Benzyl acetate	60
Terpineol	70
Cinnamic alcohol	80
Resinodour benzoin	50
C_{12}-aldehyde	1
C_{10}-aldehyde	1
Coumarin	30
Heliotropin	80
Musk ketone	50

Abd el Hajoui

	Grammes
Bergamot oil	180
Neroli oil	55
Jasmine oil absolute	15
Rose oil absolute (Moroccan)	10
Coriander oil	5
Liquid orris oil	80
Wood complex	220
Linalol	50
Cinnamic alcohol	80
Vanillin	70
Coumarin	60
Heliotropin	65
Resinodour storax	10
Resinodour benzoin	70
Musk ketone	30

Yen Pen

	Grammes
Bergamot oil	350
Ylang-ylang	60
Oak moss	15
Mace oil	10
Caraway oil	10
Cardamom oil	50
Patchouli oil	10
Clary sage oil	50
Jasmine oil absolute	10
Vetiver oil	40
Linalyl acetate L	130
Linalol L	120
Vanillin	15
Coumarin	45
Musk ketone	35

Jabberwocky

	Grammes
Bergamot oil	180
Lemon oil	60
Oil of wood complex	145
Coriander oil	60
Bulgarian rose oil	10
Oil of lavender	15
Clary sage oil	10
Jasmine oil absolute	50
Oil of orris	25
Labdanum oil absolute	15
Panaxol base	285
Ionone	5
Civet	5
Vanillin	40
Coumarin	35
Musk xylene	60

Magneto

	Grammes
Bergamot oil	180
Neroli oil	65
Rose oil	25
Vetiver oil	50
Orange oil (Guinea)	65
Sandalwood oil	25
Ylang-ylang	100
Jasmine absolute	25
Methyl ionone	160
Benzyl acetate	80
Diantax base	50
Resinodour benzoin	70
Vanillin	20
Castoreum (5 per cent.)	5
Methyl nonyl acetaldehyde (10 per cent.)	15
C_{10}-aldehyde (10 per cent.)	15
C_{10}-(?) aldehyde (10 per cent.)	10
Musk ketone	40

Kao Tsong

	Grammes
Oak moss	170
Jasmine oil absolute	50
Artificial jasmine oil	100
Vetiver oil	50
Sandalwood oil	40
Ylang-ylang	33
Rose oil (Moroccan)	10
Rose oil (Bulgarian)	20
Patchouli oil	10
Costus oil	2
Methyl ionone	100
Cinnamic alcohol	25
Phenylethyl alcohol	45
Vetiveryl acetate	30
Styrallyl acetate	10
Hydroxycitronellal	40
Linalol	40
Artificial carnation (extra)	10
Amylcinnamic aldehyde	2
Dimethylhydrocinnamyl	20
Artificial gardenia	100
C_{10}-aldehyde	5
C_{11}-aldehyde	25
Methyl nonyl aldehyde (to 10 per cent.)	5
Vanillin	20
Musk ambrette	10
Musk ketone	20

Pervenche

	Grammes
Bergamot oil	200
Geranium oil	50
Rose oil absolute	10
Jasmine oil absolute	25
Artificial jasmine oil	20
Jonquil oil absolute	10
Orange oil absolute	10
Oil of wood complex	70
Ylang-ylang	10
Artificial narcissus oil	50
Phenylethyl alcohol	50
Isoeugenol	50
Benzyl acetate	60
Amyl salicylate	50
Methyl acetophenone	20
Aurantiol	60
Artificial civet	5
Hydroxycitronellal	10
Coumarin	100
Vanillin	15
Heliotropin	20
Musk ambrette	20
Musk xylene	10
Tolu tincture	15
Storax tincture	15
Oak moss tincture	15
Tonka tincture	15
Vanilla tincture	15

Aldehyde Notes

It has been possible to make wide variations in formulæ because of the introduction of aromatic aldehydes. These materials have a tremendously powerful fragrance and assist in the rounding off of floral notes, an assistance even natural oils could not offer.

Foreign buyers considered that the French aldehyde perfumes were a revelation. One actually said: "Your first aldehyde perfume has been a French revolution against the royalty of perfume."

When "Chanel No. 5" was offered to the public, the fatty aldehydes had been known for a long time, but had practically never been used in perfumery work. Their odour was sickening, and consequently the aldehydes were not considered as possible bases for extracts. The delightful fragrance of "Chanel No. 5," and its fame, was due to the correct balancing of distinct strong floral fragrances and absolutes.

French perfumery has been dominated by the aldehyde. The great French perfumers have given a special note to their own specialty and, as a matter of fact, few extracts are produced today without an aldehydic note.

It is probably regarded as wrong in certain circles to specify ingredients for a perfume, as then perfuming and perfumery are no longer pleasures.

The aldehyde note can be described as a complete, very interesting but attenuated perfume with a particular yet real charm.

It seems as if it will continue to be popular. Will it last? It is very probable, particularly as aldehyde combinations can readily blend with the floral notes of bases, so that a new range of perfumes becomes possible.

The art of perfumery will surely develop, and with it discovery and research will move forward. Aldehyde fragrances have already won a very important position in the Golden Book of French Perfumery, and they are not likely to give this position away.

The fatty aldehydes can be blended with classical floral perfumes, but they must be used with discretion, particularly because of their great power. It is easier to use them when they have been diluted, perhaps ten times, in alcohol or a neutral solvent. Certain lactones have notes which have been imitated by synthetic materials, and these latter have had a number assigned to them and have been grouped with the aldehydes.

Grokhoff (*Parfumerie Moderne*, 1939, p. 363) recommends the use of the following:

C_8-aldehyde (octyl). It has an acrid spicy fragrance. It is not widely used but can be introduced into rose, jasmine and fancy fragrances.

C_9-aldehyde (nonyl). Has a pronounced rose odour, is a fixative which can be used in rose and orange flower notes. Is used in many compositions of aldehyde complexes used for modern fragrances.

C_{10}-aldehyde (decyl). It is difficult to define its fragrance, but it is very sweet and almost indispensable in floral compositions and eau-de-Cologne. It is found in all modern bouquets.

C_{11}-aldehyde (undecyl). It is less frequently used than the C_{10}-aldehyde. It has a strong odour, recalling slightly that of the rose. It is found in certain aldehyde complex compositions.

C_{12}-aldehyde (lauryl). It has a fatty odour which is not pleasant in the pure state, but the fragrance develops in extracts and gives them an interesting note. It is used in modern bouquets, tuberose, gardenia, lily of the valley and lilac.

C_{12}-aldehyde (methyl nonyl acetic). It is very well known and very often used. Diluted 1 : 1, it gives the bouquet of orange-flower and amber. It is largely used in the preparation of Colognes, particularly those of modern compositions.

C_{13}-aldehyde (a new aldehyde the odour of which recalls that of the rose). It can be introduced into modern compositions which contain lily of the valley and rose. Little appreciated at present, but has prospects for the future.

C_{14}-aldehyde (peach) (more correctly undecalactone). Very pronounced peach odour. It is used to impart a strong and fruity odour. It is often found in modern oriental notes, violet, jasmine and especially in fruit essences.

C_{16}-aldehyde (strawberry) (or ethyl methyl phenyl glycidate); odour of strawberries. It is very interesting because of its fruit odour, which is successfully used in certain compositions. It is found in rose hyacinth and acacia perfume.

C_{18}-aldehyde (coco) (oleic aldehyde) gives the fragrance of coconut; is rarely used in perfumery, but nevertheless gives an interesting original note to the extracts. It is generally used for its coconut aroma in fruit essences.

C_{20}-aldehyde (raspberry) (the correct formula is not known); it is possible that the commercial product is a mixture; it gives a very pronounced strong note of this fruit. Like the C_{16}-aldehyde, it can be used in perfumery.

Thus, having reviewed the aldehydes in some detail, it will be interesting to examine the combinations with each other and with both synthetic and natural products. It is known from analyses carried out on natural oils that aldehydes are to be found in almost all of the natural fragrances. The conclusion can therefore be drawn that aldehydes are necessary to bring the artificial formulations closer in odour to the natural perfumes. It is interesting to examine some possibilities.

Often C_{10}-aldehyde is found in combination with methyl anthranilate.

C_{12}-lauric aldehyde gives the bouquet of violet leaves and that of α- and β-ionone. It imparts a specified note to modern extracts with isoeugenol.

Combinations of C_{10}-, C_{11}-, C_{12}- and methyl nonyl acetic aldehyde can develop a very fashionable floral note in an extract.

Sometimes C_8- and C_{10}- aldehydes are found in jasmine compositions. C_9- aldehydes can be used in white rose; the C_8-, C_9- and C_{10}- aldehydes are often introduced into oriental rose perfumes which have a more unrestrained bouquet.

Combinations of C_{12}-, methyl nonyl acetic aldehyde, ylang-ylang, jasmine, rose, etc., essences are frequently found.

Thus the aldehydes have many applications. It should be possible to find many more compositions that could be used in perfumery if the necessary study and research are devoted to the work.

Some Aldehyde Compositions

Lily of the Valley

	Grammes
Artificial lily of the valley	200
Panaxol base or artificial opoponax	165
Labdanum absolute	100
Ylang-ylang	75
Neroli oil	60
Methyl ionone	80
Artificial jasmine (extra)	80
Jasmine absolute	60
Rose	25
Vanillin	15
Heliotropin	25
Coumarin	35
Musk ketone	50
Methyl nonyl acetic aldehyde	20
C_{11}-aldehyde	10
C_{12}-aldehyde	100

Lilac

	Grammes
Artificial lilac (extra)	250
Artificial jasmine	100
Artificial lily of the valley	100
Amber	40
Ylang-ylang	235
Artificial red rose	60
Tuberose absolute	50
Heliotropin	60
Musk ketone	30
C_{13}-aldehyde	5
C_{11}-aldehyde	5
C_{10}-aldehyde	40
Methyl nonyl acetaldehyde	20

Neroli and Rose

	Grammes
Neroli oil	100
Orange flower absolute	20
Sweet orange oil (Portugal)	140
Bergamot oil	110
Artificial lily of the valley (extra)	100
Artificial jasmine from amyl cinnamic aldehyde	110
Ylang-ylang	40
Artificial opoponax or panaxol	60
Vetiver oil	30
Heliotropin	50
Vanillin	20
Musk ketone	20
C_9-aldehyde (5 per cent.)	10
C_{10}-aldehyde (10 per cent.)	10
Methyl nonyl acetaldehyde (5 per cent.)	20

Chypre and Clary Sage

	Grammes
Clary sage	35
Oak moss absolute	50
Nutmeg oil	35
Patchouli oil	50
Vetiver oil	95
Bergamot oil	125
Concrete orris	25
Sweet orange oil (Portugal)	30
Sandalwood oil	90
Orange flower absolute	30
Jasmine absolute	30
Ionone	95
Methyl ionone	90
Labdanum absolute	40
Coumarin	25
Heliotropin	90
Vanillin	20
Musk ketone	50
C_{11}-aldehyde	75
C_{10}-aldehyde	75
Methyl nonyl acetaldehyde	50

Dihydrocarveol

	Grammes
Dihydrocarveol	150
Methyl ionone	120
Hydroxycitronellal	150
Ylang-ylang	90
Jasmine absolute	20
Artificial jasmine	120
Artificial rose	120
Artificial amber	20
Essence of tarragon	5
Heliotropin	90
Musk ambrette	15
Musk ketone	30
C_{10}-aldehyde (10 per cent.)	30
C_9-aldehyde (10 per cent.)	10
C_{12}-aldehyde (10 per cent.)	30

Lavender Extracts for the Handkerchief

The use of lavender essence in de-luxe compositions can be considered from one of two angles—*i.e.*, either as a natural or terpeneless essential oil with its original olfactory characteristics, or as linalol or linalyl acetate, which can be extracted or obtained from lavandin oil and possess little of the flower fragrance.

It is proposed to examine these alternatives in turn. The first is that in which the lavender oil plays the part often attributed to bergamot oil or to petitgrain oil, oils which are rich in linalol and its acetate. It is clear that the final fragrance will be slightly altered, as lavender oil is neither equivalent to bergamot oil nor to orange leaf oil. But such a change will be one of originality rather than one of quality.

The second much more significant alternative, yet less subject to alterations, will be that in which the ingredients play their occasional rôle in a complicated formula, or they are expressed differently, or are preponderant, to various degrees, in a symphony of fragrances. The slightly rustic note of the lavender ingredients is just as attractive as that of rosewood derivatives. The result is a slightly different yet improved fragrance.

The lavender note blends with that of "aldehyde." Each perfumer has his own preference in respect of compositions. The author's preference is known as "Cordiliere." A lavender complex follows:

	Grammes
Cordiliere (100 per cent.)	400
Lavender oil	500
Orange oil	40
Lemon oil	50
Artificial amber	10

When used at a concentration of 10 per cent. in alcohol a new aldehyde fragrance with a predominating lavender note is obtained. It can be regarded as a fragrance which men regard as pleasant. Considerable stress has been laid on the importance of the lavender, but it can be considerably reduced without seriously affecting the lavender fragrance and the general charm.

Another masculine note is given by the following formula:

	Grammes
Sandalwood oil	100
Santalene	200
Lavender oil	300
Bergamot oil	100
Caraway oil	20
Vetiver oil	35
Geranium oil	30
Rose oil (Moroccan)	8
Rosewood oil	32
Heliotropin	75
Tincture of civet	100

Lavender-like chypre fragrances are generally excellent:

Chypre I

	Grammes
Lavender oil	180
Oil of artemisia (Moroccan)	20
Ylang-ylang	70
Oak moss absolute	30
Santalene	70
Panaxol base	400
Coumarin	50
Heliotropin	80
Artificial jasmine	50
Musk ketone	50

Chypre II

	Grammes
Lavender oil	75
Linalyl acetate from lavandin	25
Linalol from lavandin	25
Panaxol base	150
Santalene	50
Coumarin	25
Heliotropin	90
Vetiver oil	35
Patchouli oil	15
Isoeugenol	30
Oak moss absolute	10
Essence of concrete orris	25
Artificial jasmine (extra)	65
Ylang-ylang oil	60
Rose oil	15
Cinnamic alcohol	80
Benzyl salicylate	70
Musk ketone	40
Musk ambrette	15

Fern perfumes from lavender are exquisite:

Fern

	Grammes
Lavender oil	250
Linalyl acetate from lavandin	200
Bergamot oil	75
Geranium oil	45
Artificial jasmine	30
Natural jasmine absolute	10
Phorax base	120
Coumarin	95
Santalene	40
Artificial rose	35
Rhodinol	40
Patchouli oil	10

The old clover formula can be rendered:

Lavender-like Clover

	Grammes
Lavender oil	250
Bergamot oil	100
Ylang-ylang	100
Benzyl acetate	70
Amyl salicylate	185
Isobutyl salicylate	125
Benzyl salicylate	70
Coumarin	60
Musk ambrette	40

The predominant note is reduced when lavandin derivatives are used instead of lavender oil. The modified preparation appears to satisfy many. In some cases it is advantageous to use lavandin constituents instead of linalyl acetate and linalol, both from rosewood, for the wood fragrances are not always rounded. This can occur with chypre perfumes. The following is not particularly lavender-like:

Chypre III

	Grammes
Linalol from lavandin	200
Linalyl acetate from lavandin	150
Vetiver	70
Santalene	30
Dianthax base or dianthine	80
Methyl ionone	100
Rhodinol	90
Coumarin	50
Oak moss	20
Sweet orange oil (Portugal)	40
Petitgrain oil (Clementier)	60
Heliotropin	50
Patchouli oil	10
Essence of pepper or spices	10
Artificial musk	40

Clementier petitgrain is obtained from orange leaves from which the "clementines" are derived. Its odour is not only different from, but is more pleasant than that of tangerine petitgrain.

If benzylidene acetone is removed from the sweet pea fragrance the latter becomes too pharmaceutical as well as too sharp even for less sensitive perceptions.

An enjoyable perfume follows:

Metamis

	Grammes
Linalyl ester from lavandin	400
Linalol from lavandin	200
Ylang-ylang	60
Vetiver oil	40
Mace nutmeg oil	20
Caraway oil	10
Cardamom oil	50
Patchouli oil	10
Clary sage	50
Oak moss absolute	15
Artificial jasmine	50
Ionone	35
Vanillin	15
Coumarin	15
Musk ketone	40

The following is a variation of an English fragrance:

Periandre

	Grammes
Linalyl ester from lavandin	400
Bergamot oil	50
Sandalwood oil	65
Santalene	100
Jasmine absolute	10
Linalol from rosewood	40
Methyl ionone	100
Coumarin	70
Heliotropin	65
Vetiver oil	35
Caraway oil	10
Rhodinol	55

Another known perfume can be rendered:

Perova

	Grammes
Linalyl acetate from lavandin	200
Ionone	100
Methyl ionone	45
Ylang-ylang	80
Vetiver oil	75
Artificial jasmine (extra)	100
Coumarin	140
Heliotropin	140
Resinoid of incense	60
Musk, artificial	60

And another:

Sunrise

	Grammes
Linalyl ester from lavandin	350
Benzyl acetate	150
Artificial jasmine	150
Methyl ionone	75
Neroli oil	15
Ylang-ylang	100
α-amylcinnamic aldehyde	50
Hydroxycitronellal	70
Rose oil absolute (Moroccan)	10
Heliotropin	80
Artificial musk	50

Robigene

	Grammes
Linalyl ester from lavandin	175
Linalol from lavandin	100
Clary sage	35
Provence Tarragon oil	15
Neroli oil	25
Vetiver oil	85
Sandalwood oil	10
Artificial rose	165
Methyl ionone	125
Artificial jasmine	85
Cinnamic alcohol	75
Coumarin	30
Vanillin	80
Heliotropin	70
Artificial musk	30

Sarpedol

	Grammes
Linalyl ester from lavandin	200
Linalol from lavandin	60
Coriander oil	5
Neroli oil	10
Sandalwood oil	100
Santalene	80
Vetiver oil	70
Concrete orris	5
Artificial jasmine	20
Moroccan rose absolute	10
Methyl ionone	90
Resinoid of benzoin	60
Cinnamic alcohol	100
Coumarin	50
Heliotropin	50
Vanillin	50
Artificial musk	40

Will these examples, among twenty others, be sufficient to convince manufacturers that by using French fragrances in greater amounts they can create good perfumes at a lower cost and at a saving to the national currency? The perfumer is naturally jealous of his inspiration. This is right, but it should not be accepted that French raw materials are inferior to exotic products. They are different and the task is assuredly to sell them.

English Formulæ for Lavender Extracts

English manufacturers have taken full advantage of the fashion in lavenders, and the low price, and have produced good products. Here are some formulæ taken from W. A. Poucher's treatise, *Perfumes, Cosmetics and Soap* (Chapman and Hall, London).

Santoline

	Grammes
Lavender oil	400
Bergamot	100
Ylang-ylang	75
Clary sage	25
Oak moss	10
Ambrette	40
Vetiver oil	50
Artificial cassia oil	50
Artificial rose oil	150
Resinodour benzoin	100

Alpine Bouquet

	Grammes
Lavender oil	400
Bergamot oil	100
Ylang-ylang	25
Clary sage	5
Rosemary	25
Jasmine	50
Ambrette	5
Geraniol	100
Ethyl phthalate	90
Resinodour benzoin	200

Fixation

Authors of other perfumery manuals have reproduced the recommendations on the technique of fixation given in the earlier formularies referred to in the introduction. The French C.I. administration have used the pre-fixation method to denature alcohol for the perfume industry. Perfumers have, therefore, been compelled to depend on synthetic musks dissolved in ethyl phthalate or benzyl benzoate. But much smaller amounts of artificial musk could have been used, as a trace of this material in an alcoholic solution renders it non-potable. They need not have compelled all to use musk, as some people dislike it.

It would be as well if some explanation of perfume fixation was given. Dr. T. Ruemelle (*Perfumery and Essential Oil Record*, July, 1948, English Journal) suggests that the fixative powers of some substances can be ascribed to adsorption phenomena. In view of the comparative lack of knowledge about them it will be of use to give at least a brief explanation.

Langmuir and Devaux have shown that there is a field of strongly attractive forces at the surface of every pure solid, even at as small a distance of 10^{-7} to 10^{-8} from it. It is believed that the molecules passing through this field are affected by it and are attracted to and stay on the solid surface, which can in this way be covered by them. Finally the surface's activity is neutralised because the attractive forces are themselves neutralised by the molecules absorbed on to the solid surface.

Such theories are based, for example, on the results of work on lubrication, as well as those in connection with "contaminated" surfaces discussed in the work on Cosmetology.

A perfume, depending on its composition, will contaminate the surface to which it is applied to different extents. The portions most strongly absorbed by this surface are those most strongly adhering to it and this in turn depends on their low volatility coefficient.

The phenomena can occur with similar compositions. Ruemelle, in reporting upon a coumarin/heliotropin mixture, points out that when the fragrance of the mixture is compared with that of pure coumarin, the fragrance of heliotropin does not decrease in the same proportion as the heliotropin is diluted. This may be explained by the formation of a monomolecular heliotropin film around the coumarin. Put otherwise, the surfaces of the coumarin crystals have a high field of attraction, and the heliotropin is adsorbed regularly on to these surfaces. Thus the coumarin cannot give off its fragrance, and it cannot be detected through that of the heliotropin.

The theory seems attractive when put forward under these conditions, but does it embrace liquid products? In this case Ruemelle's theory appears to agree with that of Arno Müller, who postulates "paragenoses," intimate, molecular associations, the odour of which is not proportional to the amount of each component. Some are actually adsorbed and no longer retain their characteristics. There still remains the question of ascertaining why one substance is more absorbent than another. It is possible that the form of the molecule plays its part, as do some physico-chemical properties—*e.g.*, the solubilities in various solvents. These are dependent on their wettability by oil or by alcohol, and it will be found that fixatives are much less soluble than the most frequently used essential oils.

Observations by different observers who are not perfumers tend to support this explanation. For example, it has been found by Clayton, Back, Jackson and Morse that polymerisation prevents crystal formation (*cf. Nature,* 1936, 138). A surface phenomenon probably explains the non-crystallisation of fatty acids (bloom) on chocolate containing lecithin (Bailey, 343). Ruemelle believes that the explanation does not wholly depend on viscosity and suggests that capillarity and other properties are worthy of study.

Whatever the explanation, he aligns himself with perfumers in his sub-division of fixatives. He divides them into auto-fixatives, pseudo-fixatives, stimulants or catalysts, and finally true fixatives. Listed among the pseudo-fixatives are some crystallisable or crystalline perfumes and he associates them with phthalic esters, benzyl benzoate, benzyl cinnamate and salicylate. Catalysts can augment certain fragrances; true fixatives have the ability to adsorb the volatile ingredients and thus delay their loss.

His list of auto-fixatives is long and unlimited. All products of low volatility are found in it, and generally they do not lower that of other fragrances. Among the products are tonquinol, vanillin, coumarin, heliotropin, benzyl isoeugenol, phenyl oxide, neroline, hydroxycitronellal, aurantiol, phenylethyl alcohol, Peru balsam, guaiacum wood oil, etc. Although the list is given as quoted, some reservations are necessary in respect to it.

Ruemelle observes that resins and gums are excellent fixatives. He attributes their value as fixatives to the considerable adsorptive effect of the colloidal materials found in the colloidally dispersed systems. It can only be a question of the interfacial activity of the high-molecular weight resin gums leading to an adsorption of the less polymerised materials. It is possible that resins, balms and like products form colloidal complexes with a low volatility, even though the materials to which they are added are volatile. Not only do they contain volatile materials, but also highly polymerised materials which are not easily distilled in steam. These high polymers have a low volatility, are more readily soluble in fats than in dilute alcohol, and in some respects are similar to resins.

The constituents of natural civet, musk and castoreum are high-molecular weight substances of a biological nature, and they vary in their volatility. Their value as fixatives is readily understood.

It is necessary to study carefully the fixation of fragrances in vehicles other than alcohol—*e.g.*, in powders, creams, milks and soaps. Datta and Tinkari believe that the best results in soap perfuming are obtained by the addition of benzyl benzoate, ethyl phthalate and even naphthalene to the essential oils. It is possible that these authors have confused fixation with succession of odours and their masking. They noticed that naphthalene covers the odour of fatty materials and that the oils in their turn cover the odour of naphthalene. This is entirely different from the adsorption by fatty oils of aromatic oils and their low evaporation as a result.

Under certain conditions essential oils are completely soluble in fatty acid esters and are not dispersed in droplet form of microscopic size, as in emulsified creams containing 20 per cent. by weight of such esters. This may account for the effect of ethyl phthalate. Sodium sulphoricinate and the ricine crystal (K) solubilise the essences and disperse them in the emulsified fatty substances as finely divided drops.

Ruemelle anticipated how important the adsorption of some fixatives by textile fibres would be, particularly in respect of their staining effect on clothes. Perfumers themselves have to reconcile the fixation of perfumes with the possible effect the fixatives they use have on materials.

Although the technique of fixation can in some ways be regarded as being standard, the possibility that new physico-chemical developments will lead to an improved fixation of oils with an elimination of the staining effects cannot be ruled out.

Specific Fixatives

Artificial musks and amber compounds are very largely used as fixatives, despite the common, slightly vulgar note they give fragrances, and it is suggested that other fixatives be employed.

A series of fixatives follow. They can be used with others that have been given or with such materials as exaltolide, civettone and other new fixatives: one for each type of floral odour.

Jasmine Fixative

	Grammes
Resinodour tolu	200
Resinodour labdanum	200
Resinodour Peru	100
Resinodour opoponax	50
Resinodour benzoin	180
Crystalline indol	50
Hydroxycitronellal	100
C_{11}-aldehyde	2
Jasmine absolute	18
Heliotropin	80
Ylang-ylang absolute	20

Orange Fixative

	Grammes
Resinodour benzoin	300
Resinodour tolu	150
Resinodour labdanum	150
Resinodour vanilla	5
Clary sage	50
Methylnaphthyl ketone	100
Neroline	50
Methyl anthranilate	100
Phenylethyl phenylacetate	50

Narcissus Fixative

	Grammes
Resinodour labdanum	300
Resinodour ambrette	200
Resinodour mastic	100
Resinodour opoponax	100
Metacresyl phenylacetate	50
Yara-yara	50
Methyl naphthyl ketone	100
Phenylacetic acid	50
Heliotropin	50

Rose Fixative

	Grammes
Resinodour olibanum	400
Resinodour orris	225
Vetiverol	75
Cedryl acetate	75
Benzyl isoeugenol	75
Phenylacetic acid	50
Citronellyl phenylacetate	50
Diphenylmethane	50

Violet Fixative

	Grammes
Resinodour labdanum	200
Resinodour orris	200
Resinodour ambrette	100
Resinodour myrrh	125
Concrete orris	75
Ethyl myristate	75
Coumarin	50
Vanillin	25
Violet leaf absolute	50

Mimosa Fixative

	Grammes
Resinodour tonka	200
Resinodour opoponax	100
Resinodour Peru	100
Resinodour tolu	100
Resinodour vanilla	100
Heliotropin	100
Hydroxycitronellal	100
Methyl naphthyl ketone	90
Cuminic aldehyde	10
Benzyl isoeugenol	50
Ethyl vanillin	25
Neroline	25

Lemon Fixative

	Grammes
Resinodour benzoin	300
Resinodour labdanum	200
Resinodour tonka	100
Isobutyl benzoate	100
Clary sage	50
Ethyl cinnamate	70
Benzyl isoeugenol	80
Neroline	35
Methyl naphthyl ketone	60
C_{10}-aldehyde	5

Orange Fixative

	Grammes
Resinodour labdanum	200
Resinodour tolu	200
Resinodour vanilla	100
Resinodour myrrh	150
Butyl cinnamate	100
Methyl naphthyl ketone	50
Methyl anthranilate	50
Methyl methyl anthranilate	50
Benzyl cinnamate	60
Clary sage	30
C_{10}-aldehyde	10

Lavender Fixative

	Grammes
Resinodour mastic	200
Resinodour storax	150
Resinodour labdanum	150
Resinodour oak moss	150
Clary sage	50
Vetiver oil	50
Heliotropin	100
Lavender absolute	100
Aldo-lavender (aldehyde)	50

Spicy Fixative

	Grammes
Resinodour incense	200
Resinodour labdanum	200
Resinodour ambrette	150
Resinodour gum elemi	100
Resinodour opoponax or clove	100
Benzyl isoeugenol	125
Cuminaldehyde	25
Estragol	25
Vanillin	25
Phenylacetic acid	25
Butyl cinnamate	25

Pine Fixative

	Grammes
Resinodour copaiba	250
Resinodour labdanum	250
Resinodour opoponax	150
Heliotropin	50
Terpeneless cypress oil	100
Oak moss absolute	50
Dimethyl hydroquinone	50
Clary sage	50
Coumarin	50

Vanilla Fixative

	Grammes
Resinodour tonka	200
Resinodour vanilla	300
Resinodour tolu	100
Resinodour labdanum	100
Butyl cinnamate	80
Ethyl vanillin	100
Heliotropin	40
Coumarin	20
Methyl isoeugenol	60

Amber Fixative

	Grammes
Civet absolute	25
Musk tonkin absolute	25
Castoreum absolute	25
Resinodour tolu	200
Resinodour labdanum	300
Terpeneless cypress oil	100
Coumarin	40
Heliotropin	60
Clary sage	90
Ethyl vanillin	35
Tincture of concrete amber	100

These fixatives make suitable, clinging fragrances for advertising cards. The fixatives are dissolved in alcohol and mixed with a 10 per cent. extract of a 100 per cent. material.

The cards are either soaked in the solution or are passed between cylinders (*e.g.*, labelling machine type) carrying the perfume.

III. VARIOUS TYPES OF PERFUMES

Floral Waxes

Some time ago there was a pronounced fashion in floral waxes packed in decorated boxes made of plastic. The high costs of alcohol, bottling and packing made these products attractive, at least to some customers, among whom may be mentioned air and land travellers and campers: people who seek to travel light. The concentrated nature of these waxes enables enough to be carried in a 5-gramme box to be equivalent to that perfume in a bottle the minimum weight of which is 100 grammes.

The waxes are usually made up of natural or artificial beeswax, ozokerite and the concretes such as are obtained by extraction with volatile solvents and from artificial complexes.

Jasmine Flowers Wax

	Grammes
Beeswax	50
Artificial jasmine	25
Concrete jasmine perfume	25

Melt all the ingredients on a water-bath and pour into the container. Solvents such as ethyl phthalate are immiscible with waxes and should not be used.

Rose Flowers Wax

	Grammes
Ceresin	35
Petroleum jelly	30
Concrete of Moroccan rose	15
Artificial rose	20

It is useful to soften the hard ceresin, but petroleum oil, which seeps out, should not be used. The mixtures may be coloured.

Lavender Flowers Wax

	Grammes
White ceresin	15
Petroleum jelly	15
Concrete lavender	50
Essence of lavender compound	20
Chlorophyll q.s.	

The concretes could be marketed either in lip rouge cases or in tubes. The former give the concretes an air of elegance; the latter are usually tin or aluminium and require a softer paste.

Soft Wax of Lilac

	Grammes
Beeswax	20
Artificial lilac	70
Concrete jasmine	10
Rose colour (q.s.)	

Any of the perfumes can be put up and sold in this pack.

SOAP PERFUMES

Soap is usually perfumed with aromatic compounds which are less expensive and less in demand than alcoholic perfumes. The examples which follow can be improved if more rounded artificial perfume materials are added. For 100 kg. of soap 500 g. to 1 kg. of the perfume is used.

Acacia for Toilet Soaps

	Grammes
Bergamot oil	100
Linalol from lavandin	100
Geranium oil	150
Atlas cedar oil	120
Anisaldehyde	200
Hydroxycitronellal	50
Methyl naphthyl ketone	50
Benzyl acetate	40
Butyl phenylacetate	50
Peru balsam	80
Musk xylene	20

Almond for Soaps

	Grammes
Oil of bitter almonds	20
Palmarosa oil	300
Terpineol	210
Anisaldehyde	20
Benzaldehyde	300
Geraniol	100
Musk xylene	50

Amber for Soaps

	Grammes
Bergamot oil	100
Peu Mou oil	50
Geranium oil	55
Patchouli oil	15
Vanillin	65
Geraniol	75
Artificial jasmine	130
Resinodour tolu	300
Resinodour orris	25
Resinodour olibanum	50
Resinodour labdanum	50
Resinodour tree moss	25
Musk ketone	15
Musk ambrette	45

Perfume: Soaps I

	Grammes
Moroccan cedar oil	200
Spike oil	200
Geranium oil	100
Clove oil	90
Lavandin oil	100
Oak moss	20
Terpineol	200
Residues	30
Resinodour benzoin S.	60

Perfume: Soaps II

	Grammes
Terpineol	250
Spike oil	200
Cedar oil (Indo-China)	200
Citronella grass oil	200
Clove oil	50
Thyme oil	20
Phenyl oxide	50
Musk xylene	30

Bouvardia Soaps

	Grammes
Bergamot oil	150
Lebanon cedar oil	60
Benzyl acetate	150
Artificial sweet pea	40
Citronellol	150
Artificial neroli	160
Amyl salicylate	100
Phenylethyl alcohol	100
Methyl anthranilate	75
Musk ketone	15

Camomile Soaps

	Grammes
Moroccan camomile oil	120
Geranium oil	300
Terpineol	340
Coumarin	40
Resinodour storax	200

Chypre I Soaps

	Grammes
American cedar oil	200
Patchouli oil	50
Vetiver oil	30
Bergamot oil	150
African geranium oil	50
Coumarin	60
Resinodour oak moss	80
Resinodour tolu	200
Resinodour labdanum	150
Musk xylene	10
Musk ambrette	15

Chypre II Soaps

	Grammes
Patchouli oil	40
Bergamot oil	70
Artificial orris	25
Cedrenol	200
Artificial rose	175
Citronellal	200
Methyl anthranilate	30
Resinodour benzoin	150
Resinodour tree moss	60
Musk ambrette	50

Chypre III Soaps

	Grammes
American cedar oil	150
Geranium oil	150
Bergamot oil	150
Coumarin	65
Artificial neroli	60
Artificial patchouli	35
Atlantone	175
Amyl salicylate	50
Artificial jasmine	60
Vanillin	5
Resinodour oak moss	75
Musk ambrette	10
Artificial orris	5
Musk xylene	10

Chypre IV Soaps

	Grammes
Compound wood oil	230
Linalol from lavandin	150
Oak moss	40
Sassafras oil	20
Labdanum absolute	20
Patchouli oil	80
Methyl cinnamate	50
Gingergrass oil	100
Ionone residues	80
Resinodour benzoin	100
Resinodour Peru	100
Musk ketone	30

Chypre V Soaps

	Grammes
Terpineol	300
Linalol from lavandin	100
Geranium oil	100
Patchouli oil	50
Oak moss absolute	100
Labdanum absolute	50
Coumarin	50
Ionone residues	200
Methyl anthranilate	20
Artificial musk	30

Chypre VI Soaps

	Grammes
Spike oil	100
Lavandin oil	200
Patchouli oil	50
Cedar oil	150
Amyl salicylate	150
Coumarin	125
Resinodour benzoin	175
Musk xylene	50

Cologne I Soaps

	Grammes
Lavandin oil	200
Citronella	200
Red thyme oil	50
Rosemary	50
Methyl naphthyl ketone	50
Methyl anthranilate	100
General residues	350

Cologne II Soaps

	Grammes
Petitgrain oil	250
Lemon oil	200
Lavandin	200
Guinea orange oil	50
Rosemary	50
Thyme oil	30
Clary sage	20
Terpineol	100
Resinodour benzoin for soaps	80
Musk ambrette	20

Cologne III Soaps

	Grammes
Citronella	200
Lavandin	200
Spike oil	100
Rosemary	80
Thyme oil	50
Orange ketone	50
Methyl anthranilate	100
Resinodour benzoin (Sumatra)	200
Musk xylene	20
Resinodour oak moss	90
Musk (xylene ?)	20

Cologne IV Soaps

	Grammes
Bergamot oil	300
Lavender oil	160
Rosemary oil	100
Linalyl acetate	100
Geraniol	120
Citral	160
Artificial neroli	80
Musk xylene	40

Cologne V Soaps

	Grammes
Rosemary oil	60
Lavender oil	120
Spike oil	40
Citronella oil	40
Petitgrain oil	120
Terpenyl acetate	250
Geraniol	200
Artificial neroli	50
Resinodour benzoin	100
Musk xylene	20

Cologne VI Soaps

	Grammes
Rosemary oil	160
Lavender oil	150
Bergamot oil	150
Guinea orange oil	100
Petitgrain oil	100
Citronella oil	100
Crystalline neroline	20
Resinodour benzoin	200
Musk xylene	20

Cologne VII Soaps

	Grammes
Bergamot oil	300
Portugal oil	150
Rosemary oil	70
Lavandin oil	150
Petitgrain oil	130
Clove oil	10
Artificial neroli	50
Vanillin	50
Resinodour tolu	80
Resinodour labdanum	100
Artificial musk	10

Cyclamen Soaps

	Grammes
Hydroxycitronellal	300
Linalol of lavandin	150
Terpineol	200
Citronellol	200
Heliotropin	50
Phenylethyl acetate	80
Musk xylene	20

Orange-Flower Soaps

	Grammes
Petitgrain oil	150
Geranium oil	100
Artificial neroli oil	250
Vanillin	10
Benzyl acetate	365
Methyl anthranilate	80
Bromelia yara-yara	20
Musk xylene	25

Fern I Soaps

	Grammes
Lavandin	250
Artificial bergamot oil	80
Artificial neroli oil	90
Moroccan cedar oil	300
Patchouli oil	30
Coumarin	60
Heliotropin	10
Amyl salicylate	70
Resinodour oak moss	90
Musk xylene	20

Fern II Soaps

	Grammes
Spike oil	120
Pale thyme oil	75
Patchouli	35
Artificial neroli oil	40
Amyl salicylate	200
Heliotropin	25
Cinnamic alcohol	60
Coumarin	100
Phenyl oxide	70
Resinodour benzoin	100
Terpineol	170

Heliotropin I Soaps

	Grammes
Heliotropin	140
Coumarin	75
Benzaldehyde	100
Vanillin	35
Artificial neroli	70
Terpineol	300
Cinnamic alcohol	100
Resinodour tolu	50
Resinodour Peru	50
Musk xylene	50

Heliotropin II Soaps

	Grammes
Algerian geranium oil	200
Lavandin	100
Oil of cloves	100
Heliotropin	100
Vanillin	50
Coumarin	50
Anisaldehyde	50
Benzaldehyde (chlorine free)	30
Resinodour Peru	100
Resinodour benzoin (for soaps)	200
Musk xylene	20

Jasmine Soaps

	Grammes
Geranium	120
Petitgrain	60
Cananga	100
Benzyl acetate	550
Methyl anthranilate	20
Linalol	120
Heliotropin	20
Neroline	10

Lettuce Soaps

	Grammes
Lavandin	350
Bergamot	250
Bitter almond oil	15
Artificial neroli	120
Geraniol	240
Musk xylene	25

Lavender I Soaps

	Grammes
Lavandin	200
Spike oil	200
Oak moss	75
Petitgrain oil (Clementier)	75
Rosemary oil	50
Wood complex	150
Lavender fractions, residue	175

Lavender II Soaps

	Grammes
Lavandin	400
Spike oil	150
Rosemary oil	100
Cedarwood oil	100
Petitgrain oil	50
Mint oil	10
Thyme oil	20
Resinodour oak moss	10
Resinodour labdanum	10
Resinodour patchouli	30

Lavender III Cola Soaps

	Grammes
Lavender oil	300
Spike oil	200
Rosemary oil	40
Rosewood oil	50
Geranium oil (Bourbon)	35
Patchouli oil	20
Red thyme oil	40
Geraniol	40
Terpenyl acetate	100
Benzylidene acetone	50
Heliotropin	60
Coumarin	30
Musk xylene	35

Lilac Soaps

	Grammes
Phenylacetaldehyde	20
Artificial rose	60
Terpineol	500
Terpenyl acetate	100
Geraniol	80
Linalol	80
Crude ionone	50
Artificial neroli	20
Heliotropin	90

Lily I Soaps

	Grammes
Terpineol	250
Linalol from lavandin	200
Artificial neroli	250
Artificial orris	100
Anethol	25
Artificial sandalwood	75
Artificial neroli	50
Musk xylene	50

Lily of the Valley I Soaps

	Grammes
Terpineol	215
Benzyl acetate	215
Linalol from lavandin	180
Lavandin	125
Phenylacetaldehyde	15
Cananga oil	100
Resinodour benzoin	150

Lily of the Valley II Soaps

	Grammes
Linalol from lavandin	400
Artificial liquid orris	200
Artificial neroli	100
Anethol	25
Artificial sandalwood	50
Artificial carnation	50
Musk xylene	25

Lily of the Valley III Soaps

	Grammes
Linalol	300
Cananga oil	160
Terpineol	200
Artificial lily of the valley	200
Artificial jasmine	100
Musk ketone	40

Opoponax Soaps

	Grammes
Resinodour opoponax	180
Artificial rose oil	60
Palmarosa	80
Patchouli oil	20
Bergamot oil	250
Artificial neroli oil	50
Sandalwood or cedar oil	135
Resinodour Peru	200
Musk xylene	25

Patchouli Soaps

	Grammes
Patchouli oil	200
Atlantone	400
Methyl salicylate	30
Cinnamic aldehyde	150
Geraniol	195
Musk xylene	25

Rose I Soaps

	Grammes
Gingergrass oil	200
Palmarosa	150
Algerian geranium oil	75
Patchouli oil	15
Geraniol	300
Eugenol	40
Phenylethyl alcohol	100
Phenyl oxide	100
Musk ketone	20

Rose II Soaps

	Grammes
Geranium oil	300
Lavandin	250
Vetiver oil	30
Citronellol	200
Phenyl oxide	20
Geraniol	200

Violet Soaps

	Grammes
Resinodour orris	400
Artificial orris	50
Ionone	65
Artificial bergamot	150
Terpineol	200
Cananga	30
Benzyl acetate	100
Methyl heptine carbonate	5

Windsor Soaps

	Grammes
Cinnamon oil	230
Thyme oil	150
Rosemary oil	75
Clove oil	75
Resinodour benzoin	150
Resinodour Peru	220
Musk xylene	25

Ylang-ylang Soaps

	Grammes
Algerian geranium oil	80
Cananga oil	400
Artificial jasmine	20
Vanillin	10
Linalol	80
Artificial ylang-ylang	175
Yara-yara	10
Benzyl acetate	200
Musk xylene or ketone	2

Lavender Perfumes for Soaps

The soap industry has found that customers like lavender perfumes. Accordingly every manufacturer seeks to surpass his competitor in the quality of his lavender fragrance. Yet it must be recognised that the perfuming of toilet soaps is difficult. Furthermore, manufacturers appreciate that results can vary not only with a particular perfume, but also with the batch of toilet chips used and its source.

Formulæ for soap perfumes can only indicate the broad paths along which success is to be found. Patience and technique will ultimately lead to it.

Some manufacturers consider that oil of lavender is insufficiently stable because of its high ester content and the possibility that the soap alkali can split the esters. Others regard this interpretation as wrong. There are certain qualities in the oil which are responsible for its pleasing fragrance, but the linalyl acetate content of the oil is not of these qualities.

Lavandin is somewhat less powerful than fine lavender oil. When it is combined with some true Provence spike, it is found to be relatively resistant to traces of alkali as well as being able to mask any fatty odours.

It is generally agreed that a combination of lavender and sesquiterpene alcohols gives a high degree of stability and alkali resistance, mainly because solid paragenoses are formed. The cedar oil fraction known as cedrenol, with its distinctly marked wood odour and uncontaminated by other odours, appears to preferable to American cedar oil, which is not only much more expensive but is mainly composed of sesquiterpenes.

The foregoing comments may be weighed when the following formulæ of Cola are modified.

Lavender I for Soaps

	Grammes
Lavender oil	525
Bergamot oil	80
Rosewood oil	100
Geranium oil	50
Rosemary oil	50
Patchouli oil	50
Clove oil	25
Coumarin	40
Musk	30
Heliotropin	50
Benzoin	25

Lavender II

	Grammes
Lavender oil	300
Spike oil	100
Rosewood oil	50
Geranium oil	35
Patchouli oil	20
Thyme oil	40
Rosemary oil	40
Geraniol	40
Terpenyl acetate	100
Benzylidene acetone	50
Coumarin	30
Heliotropin	60
Musk xylene	35

Lavender III

	Grammes
Lavender oil	100
Spike oil	400
Thyme oil	50
Citronella oil	100
Terpineol	150
Geraniol	100
Benzylidene acetone	50
Heliotropin	50

It is suggested that cedrenol should replace the terpenyl acetate and terpineol, that Moroccan cedar oil should replace the benzylidene acetone and that lavandin should replace the rosewood and bergamot.

Lavandin is an inexpensive raw material and one of the cheapest used in the soap industry. It is almost as cheap as citronella, which barely ten years ago was regarded as a cheap common product.

Odorant Fumigants

The forms in which these products are offered are cones, machine-made parallelopipeds, sticks or coils. They are used to generate pleasant fragrances, disinfectant vapours, or as insect repellents. Usually they consist of carbon and combustible cellulose materials.

	Grammes
Pulverised charcoal	600
Very fine sawdust	300
Potassium nitrate	50 to 100

These powdered products are mixed with a 2 per cent. gum tragacanth mucilage, or better still with a methyl cellulose gel in order to bind them. The perfumes show a wide variation. Resinous perfumes are largely used because they give off more fumes in use and because they do not evaporate readily. Natural or artificial fragrances can be used with the resinous materials.

The basic formula can be:

	Grammes
Combustible mixture, as above	900
Benzoin, tolu, incense, etc., resin	75
Perfume	25

By using a sawdust which will give pleasant smelling fumes—*e.g.*, cedar, larch—it is possible to reduce the amount of perfume to one-half or even lower.

Rose Fumigant

	Grammes
Combustible mixture	950
Resins from distillation	10
Colophony	10
Sumatra benzoin	10
Phenyl oxide	20

Materials which have insect repellent properties are added—*e.g.*, pyrethrum oleo-resins, artemisia oil, derris or pyrethrum flowers in the form of powder, ethyl or methyl phthalate.

Insect Repellent Fumigant I

	Grammes
Combustible mixture	920
Sumatra benzoin	20
Pyrethrum oleo-resin	5
Methyl phthalate	55

Insect Repellent Fumigant II

	Grammes
Combustible mixture	880
Lavender flowers powder	65
Pyrethrum powder	35
Derris powder	15
Oil of artemisia	5

Oriental Fumigant—Aromatic Mixture

	Grammes
Resinodour benzoin	550
Resinodour incense	300
Artificial musk residues	50
Crystalline coumarin	30
Crystalline vanillin	20
Clove oil	25
Cinnamon oil	25

Violet Fumigant—Aromatic Mixture

	Grammes
Resinodour labdanum	400
Resinodour opoponax	200
Resinodour storax	200
Total ionone	190
Methyl heptine carbonate	5
Vanillin	5

Papers for Burning

Fumigants are obtained sometimes in the form of so-called "Armenian paper." This is an unsized paper which has been treated first with 5 per cent. saltpetre solution and then with perfume. Perforation of the paper into strips can be carried out while the paper is wet if it is handled carefully, but not if machines are used. The aromatic solution is applied either by soaking the paper in the solution or by spraying it on or by coating the paper as it passes through a two-roller device. The solutions used closely resemble those used for fumigants.

Composition

	Grammes
Resinodour benzoin	300
Resinodour storax	100
Resinodour labdanum	200
Resinodour opoponax	50
Crystalline neroline	50
Artificial lilac (100 per cent.)	175
Crystalline heliotropin	100
Artificial musk	25

Not only can the quantities in the foregoing be varied, but use can be made of different perfumes.

Disinfectant Paper—Aromatic Composition

Eucalyptol
Borneol
Thymol or carvacrol
Eugenol
Cinnamic aldehyde
Resinodour tolu.

Liquids for Lamps

Methyl alcohol-burning slow combustion lamps, with plated heads, give off formaldehyde the odour of which can be masked by suitable perfumes. Resins or fatty essences cannot be used in such perfumes if they tend to dirty the wick.

Mixture for Lamps

	Grammes
Citronellol	500
Phenylethyl alcohol	100
Terpeneless geranium oil	100
Eucalyptol	100
Menthol	10
Methyl ionone	100
Eugenol	90

for 100 litres of methyl alcohol.

Fragrant Pellets for Central Heating

Central heating is very convenient but it dries the air of inhabited rooms. People cannot be persuaded to have saucers of water available in such heated rooms so that the necessary humidity can be maintained in the air. Yet quite good results occur when the air is perfumed.

Perfumes for this purpose are sold in pellets, and are intended for the water contained in a receptacle placed upon a radiator. The tablets are compressed adsorbent powders made from powdered magnesium carbonate and silica mixed with a methyl cellulose gel. The mixture is compressed into tablets in a suitable machine.

When the pellets are dry they are dipped into a perfume in which some soap has been dissolved, the soap hindering evaporation of the perfume.

Perfume for Radiators

	Grammes
Powdered soap	100
Denatured alcohol	800
Perfume (100 per cent.)	100

Immerse the dried tablets in this mixture. Alternatively, place the tablets on a sieve, pour some perfume on them and allow the tablets to dry.

Theatre Perfumes

The atmosphere of modern buildings, particularly cinemas, is conditioned. The air is drawn out, washed, reheated, humidified or dried as occasion demands. It can be perfumed or disinfected during these treatments. Buildings which do not have the necessary equipment for air-conditioning can be treated by means of diffusers, ionisers, sprays and ventilators.

Aqueous solutions of water-miscible perfumes are used. Some such solutions contain 75 per cent. by weight of absolutes. They even form stable milks.

These products are sold to schools, offices, public establishments, hospitals, clinics, etc.

Rustic Fragrance

	Grammes
Pine oil, miscible (75 per cent.)	600
Lavender oil, miscible (75 per cent.)	200
Thyme oil, miscible (75 per cent.)	180
Mint oil, miscible (75 per cent.)	20

Mountain Bouquet

	Grammes
Pine oil, miscible	500
Larch tree oil, miscible	250
Oak moss, miscible	50
Fern oil, miscible	200

Garden Bouquet

	Grammes
Rose oil, miscible	350
Lilac oil, miscible	350
Fern oil, miscible	300

Hill Bouquet

	Grammes
Siberian pine oil, miscible	600
Lavandin, miscible	100
Thyme oil, miscible	100
Pennyroyal mint oil, miscible	100
Rosemary oil, miscible	100

Floral Bouquet

	Grammes
Jasmin oil, miscible	200
Lilac oil, miscible	200
Rose oil, miscible	200
Neroli, miscible	200
Cologne, miscible	200

Provence Bouquet

	Grammes
Cypress oil, miscible	400
Lavandin, miscible	200
Thyme oil, miscible	150
Petitgrain oil, miscible	150
Orange oil, miscible	100

Antiseptic Perfume

	Grammes
Eucalyptus oil, miscible	500
Cypress oil, miscible	150
Clove oil, miscible	100
Cinnamon oil, miscible	100
Thyme oil, miscible	150

Mixtures on the lines of the foregoing can be formulated so as to meet specific requirements.

VOLATILE PERFUMES
(FOR ATOMISATION INTO THE AIR)

Perfumes intended for atomisation consist of solutions of artificial and natural compounds in deodorised kerosene. They can be atomised by compressed air.

Rustic Perfume

	Grammes
Deodorised kerosene	900
Siberian pine oil	90
Artificial jasmine oil	10

Perfume of Hills

	Grammes
Deodorised kerosene	900
Lavandin	20
Thyme oil	20
Pennyroyal oil	20
Rosemary	20
Geranium oil	20

Antiseptic Bouquet

	Grammes
Kerosene	900
Eucalyptus oil	50
Cypress oil	10
Clove oil	20
Cinnamon oil	10
Thyme oil	10

Insecticide Spray I

	Grammes
Kerosene	990
Pyrethrum oleo-resin	3
Perfume	7

Insecticide Spray II

	Grammes
Kerosene	980
Pyrethrum oleo-resin	2
Derris oleo-resin	1
Butyl phthalate	10
Perfume	7

Insecticide Spray III

	Grammes
Kerosene	980
Moroccan artemisia oil	10
Pyrethrum oleo-resin	3
Methyl phthalate	7

Perfumes for Beauty Products

Essential oils, their components and synthetic ingredients are said to have beneficial properties for the skin and mucous membranes. Such properties may account for their accepted popularity.

Yet perfumers have found it necessary to limit the amounts of perfumes they use, especially in products which are used daily. They have found that there is risk of causing irritation when the products are repeatedly used—*e.g.*, lip rouge.

A review of the beneficial properties of essential oils shows that they are, in general, antiseptic as well as healing. In addition they are said to stimulate the blood circulation and to heal such disfigurements of the skin as excoriations, cracks and crevices. Furthermore, they (the oils) assist the epidermis to defend itself against air and dust-borne micro-organisms.

Some essential oils stimulate cell growth and the consequent renewal of cells can give the skin an unattractive appearance. Examples of oils with an effect of this kind are arnica, rosemary, lavender, sage, marjoram, aniseed, coriander, fennel, visnage, etc.

English perfumers often use very dilute solutions of arnica as a homœopathic remedy with considerable success. Witch hazel exerts its effect by virtue of the small percentage of essential oils in it. Neroli oil is soothing and can be used, with great advantage, to treat the unæsthetic scars of rictus origin, particularly on the face.

Considerable discrimination is necessary in the choice of perfumes for lipsticks, lip-rouges and the like. The flavour of such perfumes is also very important, since the purpose of the lip products is to moisten as well as soften the oral mucosa. It is essential, therefore, that these perfumes have an agreeable taste even if it is not edible. Of course, regard must be had of the shortcomings of some compounds used in perfumes. Some can give rise to a burning effect because they are irritants. A good example is benzylidene acetone which, however, is used in pharmacy for its counter-irritant properties. Terpenes and terpene-rich essential oils—orange, lemon, tangerine, juniper—are likewise used. Other examples are phenyl acetic acid and benzoic acid; the latter crystallises in very sharp, fine needles. Benzyl benzoate can lead to conjunctivitis when used in eye make-up. Hydroxycitronellal and its compounds can cause unpleasant burns, and they should not be used in beauty products. Cinnamates are considered to be astringents, but they also have a caustic effect.

The phenols, particularly thymol, cause the skin to redden; the effect is less marked with eugenol. It is necessary to test carefully the effect of phenols themselves, as well as compounds containing them, unless it is decided to make no use of such materials. As mentioned earlier, they can colour the skin. Phenyl acetaldehyde is slightly irritant; cinnamic aldehyde is a vasodilator and gives a sensation of warmth. Menthol is a vasoconstrictor. In view of the cold sensation it produces on the skin when used at a concentration of 5 per cent., it is very much better to use much smaller amounts or to replace it by mint oil. It must be remembered that perfumery and beauty preparations must not contain drugs or the like in pharmaceutical amounts as they are anything but pharmaceutical preparations. Menthol is to be regarded as a medicinal product.

All in all it is very difficult to compound a satisfactory perfume for lip-rouge. It is possible to use rose bases and supplement them with terpeneless cedrat essence, jasmine and lilac essential oils. Hydroxycitronellal and phenyl acetic aldehyde should not be used. The perfume is made more pleasant with vanilla or specially sweetened amber. Synthetic musks should not be used. Too much importance should not be attached to the actual composition, provided the perfume has a good, pleasant flavour and yet is both soothing and emollient.

Perfume for Lip-Rouge

	Grammes
Terpeneless geranium oil	215
Benzyl acetate	180
Concrete essence of jasmine	215
Concrete essence of rose	75
Concrete essence of orange	75
Resinaroma of vanilla	75
Phenylethyl alcohol	105
Ethyl vanillin	60

Perfumes for Powders and Make-ups

Face powder and powder perfumes—*e.g.*, for talc—are no less delicate and, as might be expected, they bring new problems.

The so-called "powdered" odours give a very pleasing suggestion of lightness and airiness. Good perfumes should have the required properties of fineness and tenacity, but it is the fragrance of the perfume that really gives its merit.

In the past century powders were almost entirely composed of finely divided perfume materials—*e.g.*, musk ambrette, clove, Florentine orris, lemon and orange peel and ambergris. Pradal has suggested the following in a powdered form: Provence rose petals, benzoin, cinnamon bark, storax, bergamot skin, orange buds, sandalwood and angelica. By reducing them to a fine impalpable powder a powder base was obtained. It was redolent of the chosen flowers and/or exotic wood, and the fragrance is extraordinarily difficult to imitate.

The author has at one time or another suggested powdered vetiver root, heliotropin, crystalline esters, isoeugenol, coumarin, sesquiterpene alcohols and their esters, vetiveryl acetate, santalol.

There are some perfumes which have a "misty" fragrance, and it is these perfumes which enhance the feeling of airiness. Of course, the same perfume in different forms of products will give distinct shades—*e.g.*, in alcohol, oil, cream and powder. What may be very satisfactory in one vehicle is entirely unsatisfactory in another. Certainly the extract, lotion, cream and powder of a particular toilet range should not contain the same perfume. The perfume should be adjusted to suit the product in which it is used and be fashioned for it.

While handkerchief perfumes can contain a large amount of fixatives, this is not the case for lotion and cream perfumes. The powder perfumes should have the type and amount of fixatives specially adjusted.

Another difficulty that must be considered is that of oxidation so readily promoted by the finely powdered nature of the product. Clearly some essential oils and components cannot be considered for use. Oils rich in terpenes quickly become varnish or turpentine-like in smell; aldehyde perfumes lose their fragrancy power because they are oxidised to acids which often are odourless. It may be remarked that combinations of materials will undergo these changes unless they form polymers in alcohol.

Finely Divided Perfumes for Powders and Make-ups

Powder perfumes must be long lasting and resistant to oxidation, particularly as they are in mixtures charged with air. The perfumes must also suit the vehicle and must suggest a powder note. Such a note is usually obtained through heliotropin as well as perfumes with an orris note. Special fixatives, as well as artificial musk, will improve the fragrance still further. The finely powdered form results when the perfume is mixed with a highly adsorbent powder such as magnesium carbonate.

Jasmine Powder Perfume

	Grammes
Essence of artificial jasmine	100
Magnesium carbonate	700
Jasmine fixative	100
Heliotropin	80
Musk xylene	20

The jasmine essence can, of course, be replaced by an essence of lilac, lily of the valley, cyclamen, bouvardia.

Orange Powder Perfume

	Grammes
Artificial acacia or sweet pea	100
Magnesium carbonate	700
Orange fixative	100
Heliotropin	50
Musk ambrette	50

Narcissus Powder Perfume

	Grammes
Artificial narcissus, hyacinth, gardenia	100
Magnesium carbonate	700
Orris resinodour	50
Synthetic civet	50

12

Rose Powder Perfume

	Grammes
Artificial rose	100
Magnesium carbonate	650
Crystalline floranal	50
Orris resinoid	150

Lavender Powder Perfume

	Grammes
Artificial fern or lavender compound	100
Magnesium carbonate	700
Orris resinoid	50
Lavender fixative	100
Musk ambrette	50

Spicy Powder Perfume

	Grammes
Artificial carnation	100
Magnesium carbonate	700
Benzyl isoeugenol	30
Heliotropin	35
Musk ambrette	35

Perfumes for Oils

Perfumes do not readily dissolve in mineral oils. Accordingly the 100 per cent. perfume material is first blended with a vegetable oil and the perfumed vegetable oil is then mixed off with the mineral oil. In this way a clear homogeneous product is obtained.

Attention must be paid to the rancidity-promoting effect of essential oils containing terpenes or vegetable oils. To some extent this effect is countered by anti-oxidants, but at best the effect is only palliative. If terpeneless essential oils are used, then the rancidity trouble is eliminated. In view of the effect that mineral and vegetable oils have upon the fragrancy strength of the perfumes, it is necessary to use different ones from those used—*e.g.*, in powders.

Paraffin oils are frequently more difficult to perfume than petroleum oils. Solubilised castor oil or liquid compounds of fatty alcohols are useful materials to use, for they facilitate the perfuming of oils and ensure clarity without the need for filtration.

Oil Perfume

	Grammes
100 per cent. complex	200
Solubilised castor oil	500
Oleyl alcohol or ester of oleyl alcoho	300

Conclusions

It has been an object of this work to discuss formulæ, methods and technique common to the perfumery industry. This has been done so that young entrants into the art would have a clear picture of their future career. There is an undoubted shortage of perfumers in France: those who are at work are promoting and spreading the fame and glory of Parisian perfumes throughout the world. There are some who have introduced new notes. Others, sometimes working with chemists, have given their bouquets a rare originality by means of synthetics which are kept secret. The author's opinion is that there are still not enough. French perfumes have always been exported and will always be.

Perfumery can help to maintain the very high reputation for both perfection and originality that France has always enjoyed in art and in luxuries.

The fame of French products will be carried to the four corners of the world and such products will be in flawlessly designed French flasks. For the archæologists of the future the flasks will provide evidence of the dominant position French perfumery held in the world at the end of the twentieth century. It will be evidence, similar to that afforded by the large number of urns found in Cyprus, of the importance of the perfume industry in that island.

Beginners whom Nature has blessed with a delicately poised perception of smell should insist on taking up a profession in which this perception is used. They should spend several years perfecting their laboratory technique and training their olfactory senses. They should create their perfume bases with individual notes and they should have their bouquets and fragrances judged by as many women as possible. For women are experts in the matter of perfumes; they are competent assessors of the skilful blending of fragrances, of their appeal, and they point to the trends of fashion. It is true to say that an exquisite bouquet may be unappreciated by one generation simply because the current conceptions of what is pleasant in perfume may not include the perfume offered. Some years later the unaccepted perfume finds favour and becomes popular. Certainly the appropriate time must be chosen for the launch of perfumes with original notes, particularly if they are to be financial successes. This is the root of the problem.

Many a perfume already out of fashion in Paris, New York,

and London still finds very considerable favour and appeal in the provinces, in countries which are not so prone to the fickle vicissitudes of fashion, and in countries of the East. In support of this argument may be mentioned the ousting of the strong vulgar trade perfumes sold in Africa by perfumes fashionable in 1920.

Questions naturally arise as to what new countries are open to receive French products, what local tastes have to be met, what business openings are there, what terms are available and what amount of guidance is needed for buyers. The manufacturing perfumer must therefore think in terms wider than his city customers; he must think also of his subsidiary markets and must endeavour to visit them, to study their conditions and perforce appreciate their needs.

Exotic tropical flowers can offer as much inspiration for perfumers as do the flowers of Europe. Moreover their bouquets can lead to a very marked change in the likes of highly civilised countries.

It is eminently desirable that perfumers should have ample opportunity of visiting the clientele in other countries so as to acquire a first-hand knowledge of buyers' tastes as well as learning the atmosphere, particularly, of various localities. They will thus acquire the necessary background to influence the olfactory tastes of these countries and localities. It is only in this way that the newcomers to the profession will stand out head and shoulders above the many formulators who have been attracted to perfumery by its art and mystery.

The author will have achieved his aim if his work will have eased the entry into perfumery of those apprentices who are to succeed those great creators of French perfumes which have established France's reputation in this sphere.

FORMULARY OF COSMETOLOGY

INTRODUCTION

SINCE 1906 the author has consistently sought to guide the perfume industry into the now well-established directions. From about 1930 he has taken part in work which was designed to establish the principles of cosmetology. Physicians, chemists, biologists, pharmacists and doctors have had a share in the work of ascertaining, from the æsthetic point of view, the nature of the epidermal tissues, the reactions of such tissues and the action thereon of cosmetics. Patiently essential data and procedures were compiled from a host of clinical and practical trials. The series of publications which resulted have been translated into almost all the leading tongues. Moreover, they lead to the "something new" of the American specialists.

Work was almost at a standstill during the war. There was a great deal of leeway to be made up, particularly as more favourably situated overseas laboratories had made great progress through following up our ideas. Yet the work has extended still further, and French technique has regained, if not the top place, then one very near to it. Here the opportunity is taken to thank the many known and unknown helpers for their assistance and support. Some useful recipes are given in the pages which follow. As reasons have already been advanced in other publications for their development, technical considerations are not discussed.

Recapitulations and repetitions have been minimised in the order followed in the book: the formulæ develop logically from one to the next. The question of perfumes for cosmetics is not discussed, since it has been dealt with in the first part of this work.

COSMETOLOGY

Cosmetic products are designed to aid the beauty of the whole human body. It does not matter whether the beauty is that of the face, feet, hands, teeth—each is important.

The work is accordingly subdivided into parts. The first covers such specialities which aim at imparting an attractive appearance to the skin. It is essential that the normal physiological function of the skin, its health and lasting youth, should be associated with such an appearance, particularly from the cosmetologist's standpoint. Make-up is an artifice only, useful of course, but of secondary importance. Make-up products must be harmless and must be designed so that the composition will favour the vitality.

So-called holiday specialties have a place. Certainly the civilised nations who have adopted the ideas of a life in healthy freedom either at the seaside or among mountains are to be congratulated.

The chapters on products for the care of the hair, beard, and nails would have been much fuller developed had it not been for the earlier work, published by the author and his colleagues, on the *Theory of Hair*. The required information can be found in this work.*

Detergency theories as well as those concerning emulsions are to be found in E. Mahler's books; lip rouges are dealt with in *Modern Perfumery*, No. 8.

This work has been dedicated to manufacturers by the author as a source of information. Yet this book has all the elements of serious profitable manufacture.

1. *BEAUTY CREAMS*

Petroleum Jellies

Petroleum jellies are often used when a protective, physiologically inert, greasy, neutral material is required for one of the following purposes: (*a*) protective coating; (*b*) make-up remover; (*c*) vehicles for preparations containing chemical compounds which emulsions cannot tolerate, as they might break.

Natural petroleum jelly has a semi-transparent, fatty appearance. It can vary in colour from yellowish-orange to greenish-white. Both long- and short-fibred jellies are available. Hydrocarbon-soluble colours can be used to colour the jelly. Aromatic compounds which are lipophilic can be used as perfumes. The reason has already been given.

The addition of 1 to 3 per cent. castor oil, soluble in hydrocarbons, makes petroleum jellies spread readily in thin adherent polished layers. The following formula is thus obtained:

* *Théorie de la Chevelure*, Girardot et Cie Editeurs, p. 368.

	Per cent.
Pure petroleum jelly	97–92
Castor oil soluble in hydrocarbons	1–3
Perfume	2–5
Colouring matter	$\frac{1}{5,000}-\frac{1}{10,000}$

Artificial petroleum jellies are dispersions of artificial or natural waxes in jelly or paraffin (petroleum) oils. Macroscopically these artificial petroleum jellies are not unlike the natural products, but they lack their ropiness. When seen under the microscope the artificial products appear as waxy agglomerates dispersed throughout the mass. These agglomerates are separated from one another by gaps filled with oil. The syneresis they display can be readily explained on this basis. A long-fibred jelly can help to minimise this fault.

Artificial Petroleum Jelly

	Grammes
Paraffin	10
Ceresine or other wax	10
Ropy petroleum jelly	20
Petroleum oil	57
Castor oil soluble in hydrocarbons	3

Another wax of the required melting point can be used in place of the paraffin—*e.g.*, spermaceti.

Colouring and perfume as above.

Anhydrous Lano-Petroleum Jellies

Petroleum jellies have a relatively low melting point, low stability and a low adherence for surfaces. Lanolin is often added to correct these faults, despite its slight colour and very characteristic odour. It is certainly very strongly adherent. These lano-jellies will keep substances well dispersed and in excellent suspension, whereas petroleum jelly will not do so.

The following is frequently used in perfumery:

Lano-Petroleum Jelly

	Grammes
Natural or artificial petroleum jelly	70
Lanolin	30

Half quantities are commonly used by pharmacists.

By melting the two products a uniform mix can be obtained into which other ingredients can be incorporated.

Hydrated Lano-Petroleum Jellies

Petroleum jellies are hydrophobic, whereas lanoline is hydrophilic. By the addition of water to melted lanoline a homogeneous emulsion with a continuous oil phase is obtained. This property of lanolin is made use of when it is desired to prepare attractive creams. Hydrated lanolin is rarely used; lano-petroleum jelly is usually preferred.

Emulsions are obtained which are unctuous, sticky and cream or yellow coloured. They have a somewhat greasy odour which, however, can be covered by perfume. Both fatty and essential oils disperse readily in them; various materials either in solution or as suspensions can be added to the water, and the *p*H of these solutions are equal to that of the aqueous phase. The melting point can be raised so that the product is suitable for use in tropical climates.

The quantity of water varies between 15 and 35 per cent. of the total weight and rarely goes beyond 35 per cent., for even at this level the preparation tends to become "waxy": in other words, water is exuded when the cream is used. Air should not be introduced into the emulsion. The formula thus becomes:

	Parts
Lano-petroleum jelly	70
Water	30

The lano-petroleum jelly is brought to a temperature slightly above its melting point. The water, at this temperature, is added, and the ingredients are stirred until they are homogeneous.

Semi-liquid Pomade for Removing Make-up

	Parts
Lano-petroleum jelly	40
Petroleum oil	30
Water	30

Lano-petroleum jellies can be used as emulsion bases where there is a continuous oily phase. This phase may contain lipophilic substances such as vegetable or mineral oils, animal products such as purified lard, vitamin F or substances containing it and carotene. It may also contain hydrophiles such as glycol or glycerine monoesters—*e.g.*, stearates—provided they are free from alkaline salts, wetting agents or surface-active agents. These latter materials could break or reverse the emulsion. Water-soluble substances—*e.g.*, alcohol (dilute) and glycerine—can also be included.

Ointments containing Metal Salts

These products, like all continuous oily phase emulsions, can contain some alkaline earth or heavy metal fatty acid salts—*e.g.*, stearates of calcium, zinc, silver, lead, mercury and bismuth. Some of these products impart therapeutic or specifically cosmetic properties upon the preparation containing them. Alkaline-earth salts are used for the preparation of calcium or magnesium oleate ointments, zinc salts for zinc ointments. Bismuth and mercury salts are used in freckle ointments.

The following formula is for a modern calcium oleate ointment:

Calcium Oleate Ointment

	Grammes
Lano-petroleum jelly	30
Pharmaceutical olive oil	30
Calcium stearate or oleate	5
Water	35

This ointment is very stable, whereas commercial ointments are somewhat unstable.

Zinc Ointment

	Grammes
Lano-petroleum jelly	30
Vegetable oil	30
Zinc stearate	10
Water	30

Bismuth Ointment

	Grammes
Lano-petroleum jelly	30
Vegetable oil	35
Bismuth stearate	0·5
Water	34·5

Heavy metal salts are considered to be useful in homœopathy, although even allopathic medicine does not dismiss them. Preparations can readily be made in which very low concentrations of the metal salts are used.

Fatty Pomades

Hydrophilic esters can be used for the preparation of pomades. They must, of course, be odourless—*cf.* stearates and myristates—and include the mono-oleate prepared from vegetable oils, almond, groundnut, corn. Glycerine or glycol ricinoleates and isolinoleates (hydrophilic vitamin F) can also be used.

The following ingredients make up a pomade:

Special Fatty Pomade

	Grammes
Petroleum jelly	30
Lanolin	20
Fatty acid mono-ester	10
Water	40

The method of preparation is similar to that used for previous recipes. Emphasis is particularly laid upon the need for ensuring that no trace of soap or alkali—*e.g.*, triethanolamine—comes into the product. Glycerine, glycol and alcohol can, however, be used, and added to the aqueous phase.

Cholesterol-containing Petroleum Jellies

Some commercial emulsifiers are sterols, or mixtures containing them; the sterols are derived from lanolin, some of whose ingredients are regarded as both undesirable and superfluous. Pure cholesterol is on the market, and it is one of those class of substances which help to form water-in-oil emulsions. Vegetable cholesterol—phytosterol—has the same property. Absorption bases are easily prepared by taking up 2 to 3½ per cent. of cholesterol or 4 to 7 per cent. of phytosterol into a good petroleum jelly heated to 120°C. Cholesterol-containing petroleum jelly and lano-petroleum jellies can be used together.

The following formula is interesting:

Hydrated Cholesterol-containing Petroleum Jelly

	Parts
Petroleum jelly	58
Cholesterol	2
Water	40

It can be used in association with many earlier formulæ, when many variations are obtained. However, if cholesterol-containing petroleum jelly is used by itself it is very desirable to add to it some cetyl alcohol or mono-esters of glycerine or glycol absolutely free from any trace of alkaline material. This is stressed once again, as some commercial materials contain traces simply because alkaline catalysts have been used in the course of their preparation. When this is the case they are totally unsuited for use in an oily emulsion.

Make-up Removing Cream

	Parts
Cholesterol containing petroleum jelly, ropy type ..	30
Paraffin oil ..	10
Glycol monomyristate ..	10
Water ..	50

Cholesterol-containing Petroleum Jelly with Polar Compound

	Parts
Petroleum jelly ..	43
Cholesterol ..	2
Fatty acid mono-ester ..	15
Water ..	40

Forty per cent. of water can be easily incorporated into pomades containing hydrophilic esters, but it is difficult to incorporate such an amount into cholesterol-containing petroleum jellies.

It will be seen that as further instructions are adumbrated the formulæ become more and more schematic. This is in line with what has already been written. Natural and artificial petroleum jellies made surface-active or not, lano-petroleum jellies, all can be used with or without waxes, alkaline earth and heavy metal salts. The recipes could be repeated with slight variations so that there would be an impressive yet superfluous collection for somebody who has kindly and conscientiously followed the arguments.

Of course it is desirable to draw attention to the fact that the author considers a suitable stirring speed to be 60 to 80 r.p.m., provided the stirrers are wholly immersed in the paste in order to avoid occlusion of air. Such occlusion is barely perceptible with current stirrers, but it does aerate the mixture so that when the product is filled into containers it will tend to settle as it ages. The result is that the container appears to have been only partly filled and leads to a dissatisfied customer.

Other fatty emulsions, without cholesterol, can be made to contain 60 per cent. water if poly-alcohol octadecyl salts are used. The emulsion forms much more readily, so that there is no need to use colloid mills or high-speed mixers.

It is sometimes useful to reduce the amounts of petroleum products, since they are much more hydrophobic than vegetable and animal fats.

Fatty Milks

It is much more difficult to prepare fatty milks than fatty creams, since the former are liquid. Water globules are more readily taken up. The following formula gives good results:

Very Fatty Milk I

	Parts
Petroleum oil	35
Polyol octadecyl derivative	5
Water	60

Other fatty materials can be introduced.

Very Fatty Milk II

	Parts
Petroleum oil	30
Glyceryl ricinoleate	5
Polyol octadecyl derivative	5
Water	60

The milks are coloured in the oily phase as the petroleum jellies. The colouring matter is dissolved in the hydrocarbons and not in the water. Not much perfume is used, since it can act as a supplementary solvent and thereby disrupt the interfacial film. Careful attention must be paid to the possible effects of agitation and temperature changes. The aqueous phase of the milk can be stabilised with karaya gum solution.

Cold Cream

Cold creams are emulsions with a continuous oily phase. The dispersed aqueous phase is a more or less thick emulsion formed by the saponification of the wax by borax. Such emulsions are known as mixed emulsions, since they contain two opposite types. That in the aqueous phase is dispersed in the second. But as the water is not liquid in the strict sense of the word, the creams do not readily break. The amounts of wax and borax probably make them more readily saleable, and in any case these materials have always been considered to be beneficial to the skin. The cold creams can be regarded as having a gentler, more searching action than the cholesterinated petroleum jellies. The following simple formula will serve as an example:

Cold Cream

	Grammes
Petroleum jelly	15
Beeswax	15
Lanolin	5
Borax	0·5
Water	30

If the borax content is increased the emulsion type is reversed so that the continuous phase becomes water. It is therefore desirable to try to keep to the lower limit.

The term petroleum jelly includes any of the mixtures mentioned already in the chapters on petroleum, lano- and cholesterinated petroleum jellies. It even embraces mixtures of oils and fats with a consistency similar to that of petroleum jelly—*e.g.*, bacon fat, lard, coconut oil, palm-kernel oil, etc. It is desirable that the cold creams should contain small amounts of preservatives or fungicides—*e.g.*, metoxide, benzoxide, Nipagin, etc. Colouring matter and perfumes are well tolerated by cold creams.

Waxes other than beeswax can be used. Fatty acid esters—*e.g.*, spermaceti or its synthetic equivalent, cetyl stearate—can be used in the formula. The following is cast on the lines of an English cold cream. Petroleum jelly, as mentioned before, is a generic term.

English Cold Cream

	Parts
White petroleum jelly complex	40
Beeswax	10
Spermaceti	5
Lanolin	5
Fatty acid mono-ester	15
Water	15
Antiseptic q.s.	

American Cold Cream (*after F. Chilson*)*

	Parts
Glyceryl monostearate	15
Lanolin	3
Mineral oil	14
Glycerin	3
Petroleum jelly	2
Perfume	0·5
Water	62·5

Cetyl or oleyl alcohol can be used. Both are hydrophilic and assist the aqueous phase dispersion. Soya or egg lecithin can be in-

* Francis Chilson, "Modern Cosmetics," *Drug and Cosmetic Industry*, New York.

corporated, provided sufficient preservative is used or the product is immediately used. These phospho-lipids are very good culture media for moulds. Nutritive properties can be given to the cream by vegetable oils and animal fats.

Cold Cream with Animal Fat

I

	Parts
White wax	15
Benzoinated lard	50
Lanolin	9
Distilled water	24·5
Borax	1
Perfume	0·5

II

Tallow and lard substances	30
Lard oil	25
Cetyl alcohol or spermaceti	5
Cholesterol	2·5
Borax	0·5
Water	37

Vegetable Cold Cream

	Parts
Odourless coconut oil	30
Olive oil	20
Almond oil	10
Beeswax	5
Borax	0·5
Water	34·5

Mixed Cold Cream
(*after F. Chilson*)

	Parts
Sesame oil	42·5
Lanolin	4·5
Beeswax	15·5
Spermaceti	6
Borax	1
Water	30
Perfume	0·5

Cold Cream Complex

	Parts
Glyceryl monostearate	10
Lanolin	3
Groundnut oil	15
Hydrogenated whale oil	25
Glycerine	5
Beeswax	5
Borax	0·3
Water	36·7

Cold Cream with Triethanolamine (after F. Chilson)

	Parts
Beeswax	18
Petroleum oil	16
Lanolin	5
Stearic acid	3
Triethanolamine	0·5
Glycerine	8
Water	49
Perfume	0·5

English formulæ usually contain 30 per cent. or less water.

The examples can be multiplied *ad infinitum*. It is not useful to do so. As mixed emulsions are involved, "water phase" emulsion ingredients can be chosen to be incorporated into the already prepared oil phase.

Emulsions with a Continuous Water Phase

These preparations are termed vanishing creams by the English. They leave no traces on the skin if after application they are rubbed in, provided a thin layer is applied in the first instance. They have distinct skin penetration properties and, moreover, their *p*H corresponds to the physiological *p*H. There is a great demand for them. They can be easily prepared and their manufacture offers no risk, particularly since E. Mahler elucidated their ageing behaviour. A considerable number of preparations of this type will change their texture as they age, unless some specific ingredients—*e.g.*, gelling agents—are used to prevent the crystallisation of the fatty acids. Modern creams based on triethanolamine are subject to this shortcoming, but nevertheless they are interesting, since they contain little soap and their *p*H is low.

Stearate Creams

The early stearate creams contained large amounts of glycerine, and they had the hydrating properties needed by skins exposed to south winds and by the inhabitants of hot, arid regions. They are still in demand. If they could be aerated like egg-white when beaten, people would be satisfied with softer products. Sodium or ammonium stearate creams can be aerated so that their volume is increased. Some manufacturers have made creams with a density as low as 0·38. These whipped creams are prepared in machines in which the stirrer, with several blades, rotates at great speed. Each blade introduces air into the cream as it passes through the product.

Creams Based on Sodium Stearate

I

	Grammes
Stearic acid	22
Glycerine	65
Caustic soda	0·8
Water	13

II

Stearic acid	12
Geleol (gelling agent)	4
Glycerine	60
Sodium hydroxide (36°)	2·5
Water	21·5

The soda can be substituted by its equivalent of carbonate, particularly if an aerated product is desired. The carbon dioxide evolved will assist the process of aeration.

Cream Based on Potassium Stearate

	Grammes
Stearic acid	20
Glycerine	40
Caustic potash	0·9
Water	39

Creams Based on Ammonium Stearate

Fatty or mineral oils can be used in all these preparations, if non-aerated creams are wanted. The foregoing formulæ can be used for ammonium stearate creams.

I

	Grammes
Stearic acid	20
Glycerine	10
Petroleum oil	10
Olive oil	5
Ammonia (21°)	3
Water	52

II

Partially saponified ammonium stearate	15
Hydrine (gelling agent)	2
Glycerine	45
Water	43

The creams are subject to mould growth if their glycerine content falls below 50 per cent. The preservative must be well chosen, like the perfume.

Creams can be prepared with self-emulsifying monostearates. If spermaceti is added, care must be taken. Cetyl alcohol, a constituent of spermaceti, is hydrophilic, improves the emulsion, and can therefore be used instead.

Cetyl Alcohol Cream

	Grammes
Stearic acid	18
Cetyl alcohol	5
Sodium or ammonium carbonate	2
Glycerine	35
Petroleum oil	5
Water	43

Gum can be used to gel the water phase. In this way the amount of fatty acids can be reduced without reducing the greasy nature.

Tragacanth Cream

	Grammes
Stearic acid	16
Glycerine	30
Petroleum oil	5
Caustic potash	0·6
Gum tragacanth	2
Water	46·4

The cream can be gelled with monoesters of glycol and glycerine, and this allows other ingredients to be added—*e.g.*, petroleum jelly, cacao butter, castor oil, lecithin, sulphonated oils, soluble colouring matter, pigments, etc.

Gelled Cream

	Grammes
Stearic acid	10
Glyceryl monostearate	10
Glycerine	10
Castor oil	5
Lecithin	1
Petroleum oil	10
Caustic potash	0·2
Water	53·8

Triethanolamine Creams

The *p*H of these creams is of the order of 8·3, and is due to the hydrolysis of the soap formed by the combination of stearic acid and alkali. The *p*H is too high for beauty care. The apparently lower *p*H of the high glycerine creams is brought to its real value when the creams are diluted with water. Triethanolamine is now the alkali of choice, as its soaps have a lower *p*H, about 7. But the triethanolamine soaps are soft and become brown in time. It is better to use partially saponified triethanolamine stearates prepared by various manufacturing specialists. They have the advantage of not yellowing, and firmer creams can be made.

Cream Based on Triethanolamine Stearate

	Parts
Special triethanolamine stearate	18
Glycerine	5
Petroleum oil	8
Water	74
Preservative	1

This simple formula is used almost exclusively for shaving cream. The emollients used (glycerine and oil) are at a minimum and are insufficient for the normal care of the skin. Other materials can readily be added to triethanolamine creams as they are to other stearate creams. In order to minimise changes in the texture of creams in which triethanolamine is the alkali used, it is desirable to gel them and so prevent crystallisation of the large excess of stearic acid dispersed throughout the cream.

Gelled Triethanolamine Cream

I

	Grammes
Special triethanolamine stearate	9
Hydrine (gelling agent)	9
Glycerine	10
Petroleum oil	3
Vegetable oil	5
Water	64
Preservative *q.s.*	

II

Special triethanolamine stearate	12
Geleol	10
Glycerine	20
Metoxide	0·2
Perfume	0·3
Water	52·5

Pearly creams are those in which the stearic acid is allowed to crystallise. This crystallisation leads to a softening of the cream's texture.

Titanium oxide, a white pigment, can be added to stearate creams. It imparts a fine brilliancy to the skin. Such pigmented creams form a base for hand preparations.

Hand Cream

	Grammes
Special triethanolamine stearate	10
Glycol monostearate T.G.	9
Glycol	4
Groundnut oil	3
Water	71
Titanium oxide	3
Antiseptic and perfume *q.s.*	

Zinc oxide, alkaline earth and metal oxides must not be added to stearate creams, since they can combine with the free stearic acid to form fatty acid salts and possibly to reverse the emulsion. Cholesterol and other materials used in the continuous oily phase emulsions are best avoided in such creams.

Cream with Physiological pH (pH 7)

	Grammes
Cetasol	18
Lanolin	1
Almond oil	1
Petroleum oil	1
Glycerine	20
Antiseptic and perfume	1
Water	58

Fatty Face Cream

	Grammes
Triethanolamine stearate	13
Glycol monomyristate	6
Cocoa butter	2
Olive oil	1
Water	78
Perfume *q.s.*	

Beauty Milks

Beauty milks are readily prepared by diluting self-emulsifying fatty acid esters.

Glyceryl monostearate T.G. gives a thick milk at a concentration of 3·5 per cent. in water and a thin milk at 1·7 per cent. to 2 per cent. The stearate is melted and a portion of the water, at 95°C., is added. The mix is stirred as it cools and when cold is diluted with the remaining water.

Monomyristates, which are softer than the monostearates, yield milks which, at a like viscosity as milks formed with stearates, contain more fatty materials and are more active dermatologically.

For example, 8 parts of monomyristate T.G. are melted in

26 parts distilled water, and the preservative (0·1 of sodium phenaseptate) is added. Three grammes of petroleum oil are added and finally the perfume. When the cream is cold, 63 grammes of water are added.

Make-up Removing Milk (English)
(after Ralph G. Harry)

	Parts
Petroleum oil	10
Triethanolamine stearate	4·8
Witch hazel	35·2
Distilled water	50
Preservative *q.s.*	

Make-up Removing Milk (American)
(after de Navarre)

	Parts
Triethanolamine stearate	7
Petroleum oil	29·06
Self-emulsifying glycol stearate	0·5
Beeswax	0·05
Stearic acid	0·40
Water	63
Perfume *q.s.*	

Carbohydrate Creams

These creams form a large cosmetic class. The glycerinated starches with zinc oxide are excellent products for dehydrated skins and for use in dry countries. The amphoteric nature of zinc oxide makes it very useful for the variations in the acidity or alkalinity of the skin.

Glycerinated Starch

	Grammes
Starch	7·5
Water	7·5
Glycerine	85

Glycerine/Zinc Oxide Cream

	Grammes
Glycerine	79
Rose water	10
Starch	6
Zinc oxide	5
Perfume *q.s.*	

Moisten the starch with water, add the glycerine, and heat to 120°C. until a paste is formed. Add zinc oxide and finally perfume. The starch is sometimes replaced by gum mucilage. As a rule, mucilages are only added to stearate creams.

Agar-containing Stearate Creams

	Grammes
Triethanolamine stearate	12
Glycol stearate	5·5
Agar	0·5
Water	82
Antiseptic and perfume *q.s.*	

Gelatine-containing Stearate Cream

	Grammes
Glyceryl monostearate T.G. self emulsifying	14
Cetyl alcohol	4
Gelatin	0·6
Water	81·4
Antiseptic and perfume *q.s.*	

Homogeneous viscous milks are obtained when the water phase is gelled, the gum acting as a protective colloid. Gum karaya is mainly used.

Gelled Milk

	Grammes
Gum solution, 2 per cent.	50
Hydrophilic oil	35
Petroleum oil	13
Ammonium lauryl sulphonate	2

Cleansing Creams

All modern wetting agents are contaminants for emulsions with a continuous water phase. Thus the ammonium or triethanolamine soaps of the preceding sections can be replaced by sulphonated fatty alcohol salts or substitutes.

As they have detergent properties, such materials can be used to make creams which function as cleansing or make-up removing preparations. They can be readily prepared and, in addition, their *p*H is low. When the wetting agent is used at a high concentration the creams tend to lather on the skin—*i.e.*, they rub out white before they penetrate into the skin.

Cleansing Cream

	Parts
Special triethanolamine stearate	10
Stearic acid	6
Glycol monomyristate	4
Sodium lauryl sulphonate	3
Groundnut oil	5
Glycerine or glycol	8
Water	64
Antiseptic and perfume	*q.s.*

These creams, as others containing less than 35 per cent. glycerine, must be filled into tin or tin-coated lead tubes. Sulphonated creams are occasionally too acid for varnished aluminium tubes to be used.

Antiseptic Creams

For medical and like purposes antiseptic cleansing creams, which are more pleasant than petroleum jellies and more harmless than soaps, find a use—*e.g.*:

	Parts
Stearic acid	12
Glyceryl monostearate	8
Sodium lauryl sulphonate	3
Glycerine	10
Oil	3
Hydroxyquinoline sulphate	1
Chlorothymol	0·5
Sodium parahydroxy benzoate	0·5
Water	62

Creams with Fruit Juices

Unlike soaps, lauryl sulphonates and their substitutes are unaffected by acids. Thus creams with a *p*H below 5 can be made by emulsifying stearic acid, fatty alcohol-cetyl-, mono-esters of fatty acids with wetting agents. Sterile fruit juices can then be added.

	Grammes
Stearic acid	14
Pure glycol monostearate	6
Sodium lauryl sulphonate (30 per cent.)	3
Sterile lemon juice	20
Lemon perfume compound	0·5
Antiseptic	0·5
Water	46

Despite the use of antiseptics, etc., it is not easy to preserve the creams. The creams can only be marketed in jars or tubes made of tin or tin-coated lead. Aluminium tubes are unsuitable.

Various Creams

A wide range of materials can be used in the sulphonated alcohol emulsions. It has not yet been completely established that the daily or repeated use of substances as active as the sulphonates is entirely safe. Products for special use can be prepared:

Astringent and Deodorant Cream

	Grammes
Stearic acid	10
Glycol monostearate T.G.	8
Sodium lauryl sulphonate (30 per cent.)	4
Formaldehyde	1·25
Hydroxyquinoline sulphate	1
Preservative	0·2
Glycerine	5
Water	71·55

Analgesic Cream for Massage in Cellulitis

I	*Grammes*
Stearic acid	10
Geleol	9
Sodium lauryl sulphonate (30 per cent.)	3
Menthyl salicylate	1
Orange flower water	77

II	
Triethanolamine stearate	13
Glycol monostearate T.G.	7
Scuroform	1
Olive oil	9
Water	70
Antiseptic, preservative and perfume	*q.s.*

Camphor Cream for Massage

	Grammes
Self-emulsifying glycol stearate	12
Stearic acid	5
Petroleum oil	3
Camphor	0·5
Antiseptic and perfume	0·5
Water	79

Menthol Cream for Massage

	Grammes
Glyceryl monostearate T.G. (self-emulsifying)	12
Glycerine	3
Oleo-cetyl alcohol	5
Titanium oxide	1
Menthol	0·1
Eucalyptol	0·1
Antiseptic	0·1
Lavender oil	0·2
Water	78·5

Vitamin or Hormone Creams

Vitamins and hormones can only be used in beauty products by pharmacists, according to the law. Thus pharmacists alone have the right to sell these kinds of products provided they are adequately labelled. The cosmetician logically can use these materials when they are introduced as part of the raw materials he uses—*e.g.*, halibut, fish-liver, avocado and olive oils. The quantitative or biological evaluation of the active content is misleading, particularly at the dosage level of 50 to 100 International Units per gramme. There is no proof that they do not lose their chemical individuality with the result that they diminish in activity. The most undesirable feature of all is that the perfumer-cosmetician is prohibited from either advertising or mentioning vitamins, etc., on the label.

The author has frequently recommended provitamin A or carotene. Its action is known, and as it is not a vitamin its use is not prohibited. It is a tonic and an anti-infection agent. That it acts on the lymphatic system is evidenced by the disappearance of bags under the eyes and wrinkles. Carotene remains active in purely fatty substances, but slowly decreases in activity in continuous oil phase emulsions and rapidly in creams with a continuous aqueous phase. It can be recommended for:

I	*Grammes*
Anhydrous petroleum jelly containing cholesterol	98
Oil-containing carotene	2

A concentrated odourless halibut oil can be used.

II	*Grammes*
Hydrophilic petroleum jelly	50
Vitamin-containing oil (25,000 I.U.)	3
Water	47

III	
Lano-petroleum jelly	70
Avocado or olive oil	20
Vitamin-A concentrate	3
Water and alcohol	7

Some biological extracts such as those of tissues or organs have æsthetic possibilities. They are best made use of in beauty salons, where they can be used unmixed or mixed with creams immediately before use. The application of such a cream is followed with a massage using a penetrating cream. The extracts are supplied in ampoules. Extracts so supplied include special physiological and hæmopoietic sera, embryo extracts and fruit juices. These products must be used with some discretion and with a lack of publicity. Vitamins and synthetic hormones, in strictly controlled amounts, can likewise be used.

Creams for Special Treatments

For Breast Complaints

	Grammes
Resinodour mastic	0·3
Resinodour asafœtida	0·3
Resinodour opoponax	0·3
Jasmine oil	0·2
Carnation perfume compound	0·4
Hydrated cholesterinated lano-petroleum jelly	98·5

For Scurf and Perlèche

	Grammes
Acid cream with ketasal (1·9 per cent.)	96·5
Dissolved sulphur	2·8
Cinnamon oil	0·2
Lavender oil	0·5

For Skin Hardening

	Grammes
Zinc stearate	5
Cold cream	93
Concentrated halibut oil	1
Carotene oil	1

Sulphur Cream for Acne and Seborrhœa

	Grammes
Solubilised sulphur	3
Carotene oil (3,300 I.U.)	0·5
Lecithin	0·5
Menthyl salicylate	0·5
Geranium oil	0·5
Lavender oil	2
Borneol	0·5
Ketasal	20
Water to	100

Coloured Foundation Creams

These comprise pigment loaded fatty creams which, because of their low water content, allow more or less greasy make-ups and sufficiently liquid glycerinated creams or creams in which the pigment can be uniformly distributed. The latter class are the more popular.

The creams with polyol stearates are particularly recommended:

I

	Grammes
Glycerinated stearate cream	70
Talc	20
Titanium oxide	5
Pigment	5
Preservative and perfume *q.s.*	

II

	Grammes
Triethanolamine stearate cream	60
Glycol	20
Titanium oxide	5
Pigment	15
Preservative and perfume *q.s.*	

De Navarre, in his recent work,* gives a new formula.

III

	Grammes
Talc	40
Glycerinated starch	10
Sorbitol laurate	10
Zinc oxide	20
Sorbitol syrup	3
Mineral oil	1
Water	16
Colour, perfume and antiseptic *q.s.*	

There are very many such preparations. There will be more given in the chapter on these products.

Shaving Creams

Shaving creams are emulsified forms of shaving soap, and are usually in flexible tubes. As saponification is usually carried out with a dilute lye, it is advisable only to use easily saponified oils. The cream contains about 33 per cent. fatty acids. The latter is due to the excess stearic acid. Advantage is taken of the property that super-glycerinated or glycol-containing soaps have of remaining soft for such creams.

I

	Parts
Coconut oil	18
Stearic acid	16
Glycol monomyristate T.G.	3
Glycerine	12
Caustic potash	6·8
Water	56·2
Perfume *q.s.*	

II

Palm-kernel oil	6
Coconut oil	6
Stearic acid	25
Lauryl sulphonate (30 per cent.)	5
Caustic potash	7
Glycerine	15
Water	36

English manufacturers use borax or boric acid with an excess of alkali. The batch is stirred as much as possible, yet avoiding

* M. G. de Navarre, *The Chemistry and Manufacture of Cosmetics.* Van Nostrand Co. New York.

aeration, which will give a foamy product liable to decrease in volume.

Earlier a formula was given for a brushless shaving cream based on triethanolamine stearate. The formula can be modified by making use of a gelling agent which makes possible a reduction in the amount of stearic acid used.

Lauric acid soaps remain liquid in the presence of an excess of alkali. This property is used to mix such soaps with liquid oils —*e.g.*, olive and groundnut. When the glycerides have been saponified the excess alkali is taken up by fatty acid.

2. *COSMETIC SPECIALITIES FOR HOLIDAYS*

Certain cosmetic preparations are indispensable for both winter and summer holiday makers who spend their holidays on mountains or at the seaside. Pride of place must be given to—

Products against Sunburn

All products which allow prolonged exposure to ultra-violet rays at the beach or on the mountains come into this class. Such rays should give rise to a natural tanning of the skin and no burns. Some products should heighten the illusion of browning after the holiday resort has been reached. Classes of anti-sunburn preparations are lotions, oils, creams, etc.

Sun-Tan Lotion

The simplest sun-tan lotion consists of an aqueous solution of a brown colour.

I	*Parts*
Soluble brown colour	5
Floral water	95

Alcohol can be added to the water. Insoluble pigments can be mixed in, and in order to increase the wetting properties for an already greased skin a wetting agent may be added.

II	*Parts*
Soluble brown colour	4
Dark ochre pigment	5
Sulphonated alcohol (30 per cent.)	1
Alcohol 20°	90

A sun-screen can be used in the lotion.

III	Parts
Lotion as above	95
Alcohol solution of tannin	5

In order to improve the adherence gum may be used.

IV	Parts
Gum karaya	2
Alcohol 90°	15
Glycerine	5
Citric acid	0·75
Quinine sulphate	3·25
Perfume, colour and water *q.s.* to	100

After a long sun bath it may be advisable to stimulate the blood circulation by a counter-irritant lotion.

After-Bath Lotion

Alcohol	1 litre
Eau-de-Cologne essence (not terpeneless)	20 grammes
Cinnamon oil	4 ,,
Oil of pale thyme	6 ,,

Sun-protective Oils

Sun-protective oils are preferred to the lotions. They aid tanning and diminish the danger of burns and erythema. A vegetable oil is preferred, and it can be blended with a "film-activated" mineral oil—*i.e.*, a hydrocarbon soluble castor oil. For example:

I	*Grammes*
Fat-soluble sun screen	5
Vegetable oil	50
" Film activated " mineral oil	45
Bergamot oil	*q.s.*
Colour	*q.s.*
Anti-oxidant	*q.s.*

There are various types of sun-protective products. Some are optical screens (β-methyl umbelliferone, methyl æsculin), others (menthyl and bornyl salicylates) are, at one and the same time, filters and physico-chemical agents. These agents can halt the oxidation/reduction tendency. Yet others (pigments) are simple physical screens and absorb the rays of light. Quinine oleate is used in England.

II

	Grammes
Quinine oleate	3·5
Groundnut oil	46·0
Almond oil	50·0
Perfume	0·5
Colour *q.s.*	

III

Menthyl salicylate	5
Vegetable oil	20
Film activated mineral oil	72
Methyl parahydroxy benzoate	0·2
Perfume } for sun protection	0·3
Colour } for sun protection	2·5

An anointing oil for use after a sun-bath can be prepared.

Bath Oil (Anointing)

Vegetable oil	1 litre
Pale thyme oil	1 gramme
Cinnamon oil	1 ,,
Clove oil	1 ,,
Garden sage oil	1 ,,
Bergamot oil	8 ,,

Sun-protective Creams

The bottles holding sunburn oils are liable to break, and when they do the dangerous pieces of glass can litter roads and beaches. Creams and other emulsions marketed in collapsible metal tubes are free from this danger.

Petroleum jellies, light-coloured preferably, lano-petroleum jellies, or emulsions of the types already described in the appropriate places form this class.

Petroleum Jelly Sun Protective

I

	Grammes
Amber petroleum jelly	86
Lanolin	6
Insoluble brown pigment	5
Menthyl salicylate	2·5
Perfume	0·5

Should pigment-screens be used in large amounts, then either a cholesterinated petroleum jelly, or a cold cream with glycerine and oil, or a cream based on a stearate derivative of polyhydric alcohols should be used.

II

	Parts
Lano-petroleum jelly	70
Mineral oil	20
Sun screen (umbelliferone)	3
Pigment, brown and scarlet	7
Perfume *q.s.*	

III	*Parts*
Cholesterinated petroleum jelly	45
Menthyl salicylate	5
Alcohol	10
Water	40
Perfume and colouring matter *q.s.*	

IV	*Grammes*
Glycerinated cold cream	80
Methyl aesculin	3
Sun-coloured titanium oxide	15
Lavender perfume and antiferment	2

Ski Creams

The creams intended for use on mountains and during ski-ing in spring must be much more effective than those used on the beach. The amounts of sun screens must perforce be increased, and combinations of various means of protection must be used.

	Parts
Cholesterinated lano-petroleum jelly	65
Methyl aesculin	3
Menthyl salicylate	5
Titanium oxide	8
Dark lacquer	18
Lavender perfume	1

A bronze-brown pigment is often appreciated. Of course, if it is possible, two shades of colour should be available for different skins. The inert material used should be sufficient to prevent the sun's rays from reaching the skin. The product's melting point should be such that the preparation will not be affected by the rays.

Ointments for Sunburn

Creams, preferably acid, should be available for the treatment of erythema and of burns.

Ointment for Burns

	Parts
Emulsion of cetasal (20 per cent.)	95
Halibut oil	2
Carotene oil	2
Lavender oil	1

Ointment (Refreshing) for Erythema

	Parts
Emulsion of cetasal	95
Menthol	0·5
Bornyl salicylate	2·5
Carotene oil	2·5

Creams for Sports

Sports devotees should have at their disposal a cream suitable for dressing burns, bruises, ecchymoses, sprains, etc.

American Formula

	Parts
Zinc phenolsulphonate	2
Glycerine	5
Hydrated lano-petroleum jelly	93

Arnica Cream

	Parts
Cetasal emulsion (20 per cent.)	95
Arnica tincture	4·5
Petitgrain oil (tangerine)	0·5

A massage after a tiring excursion is often beneficial:

Massage Cream

	Parts
Cetasal	20
Hexose	10
Vitamin F	5
Carotene oil	5
Wild thyme oil	1
Water q.s. to	100

Ointment against Cramps

	Parts
Cetasal	20
Coconut oil	5
Vitamin F	5
Essence of camomile M	1
Vitamin B_3	0·1
Water *q.s.* to	100

Ointment against Chilblains and Acrocyanosis

	Parts
Anhydrous lano-petroleum jelly	50
Coconut oil	10
Borneol	1
Rosemary oil	0·1
Cinnamon oil	0·2
Lavender oil	0·2
Tansy oil	0·1
Water q.s. to	100

Marine Cream—Against Mist, Fog, etc.

A protective cream is necessary for ocean-going travellers, swimming, rowing and other nautical pursuits, whereas a hydrating cream is necessary on the southern beaches.

I

	Parts
Cholesterol-containing complex	70
Witch hazel	30

The vasomotor power can be heightened by the following in chills and contests.

II

	Parts
Hydrophilic petroleum jelly	50
Clary sage water	47
Ceylon cinnamon oil	1
Artificial carnation oil	2

Foot Cream

Walkers, ramblers, climbers need a cream for application to their feet:

	Parts
Cetasal	12
Lanolin	10
Castor oil	5
Lavender oil	1
Antiseptic	1
Water *q.s.* to	100

Cleansers

The repeated daily use of fatty products such as whale oils demands efficient rapid cleansing which ordinary soap does not usually provide. Solutions of wetting agents are used preferably.

Make-up Remover

	Grammes
Sodium sulphoricinoleate	10
Sodium laurylsulphonate	3·5
Perfume	0·5
Water	86

Hydrating Make-up Remover

	Grammes
Glycerol or glycol	30
Lauryl sulphonate liquid	5
Camphorated alcohol	2
Orange flower water	50
Distilled water	13
Colour	*q.s.*
Perfume	*q.s.*

Milk for Removing Make-up

	Grammes
Hydrophilic petroleum oil	50
Glyceryl ricinoleate	10
Sinopon	3
Water	37

Water for Removing Make-up

	Grammes
Glycol or glycerine	30
Solution of sulphonated alcohol	5
Camphorated alcohol	2
Orange flower water	63
Colour	*q.s.*

ANTI-INSECT PREPARATIONS

Many districts in France are still infested with stinging insects. French tropical colonies are also insect infested, and living there is frequently made unbearable by these parasites. There will always be a welcome for specific preparations against mosquitoes.

Protecting Cream

	Parts
Cetasal	20
Petroleum oil	5
Dibutyl phthalate	5
Citronella essence	1
Water *q.s.* to	100

Protecting Cream

	Parts
Butyl phthalate	30
Benzyl benzoate	20
Essence of artemisia	1
Lavender oil	0·5
Triethanolamine stearate	10
Hydrine	10
Water *q.s.* to	100

Cream with D.D.T.

	Parts
Triethanolamine stearate	10
Glycol monostearate T.G.	8
Petroleum oil	5
D.D.T.	5
Pyrethrum oleoresin	0·02
Water *q.s.* to	100

Cream for the Prevention and Cure of Insect Bites

I	*Parts*
Cream based on triethanolamine stearate	98·5
Essence of Moroccan artemisia	0·2
Menthyl salicylate	0·5
Butyl phthalate	0·3
Lavender oil	0·5

II

	Parts
Cream based on triethanolamine stearate	98·5
Menthol	0·25
Bornyl salicylate	0·5
Camphor	0·25
Essence of pennyroyal	0·5
Antiseptic	*q.s.*

3. *ROUGES*

Make-ups comprise various creams containing colours, and they are usually filled into bowls or jars. The technique used in lip rouges could readily give inspiration for new rouges. Anhydrous make-ups can readily be prepared from petroleum oils. They spread well, are very shiny after application, are useful for eyelashes and as a theatrical make-up. The group includes also fatty make-ups emulsified with lano- and hydrophilic petroleum jellies, as well as those based on cold cream or stearate or glycerine creams. Dry rouges, powder rouges, and compact rouge are also made.

The lakes used to obtain the desired colour must be fast and unaffected by water. Bismuth salts, as well as white lead, must not be used.

Pastel shades usually contain titanium oxide.

Anhydrous Fatty Rouge

	Parts
Cholesterol-containing complex ..	90–95
Lakes and white pigment	10–5

Adherent Fatty Rouge

	Parts
Lano-petroleum jelly complex	90–95
Lakes and white pigment	10–5

Hydrated Fatty Rouge

	Parts
Hydrophilic petroleum jelly (with 30 per cent. water)	90–95
Lakes and white pigment	10–5

Cold Cream Rouge

	Parts
Wax cold cream	70
Hydrated lano-petroleum jelly	20
Lakes and pigment	10

Glycerine-containing Rouge

	Parts
Stearate cream with 33 per cent. glycerine	88
Lakes and pigment	12

The covering power of the colours determines the amount used. It is said that 2 to 5 per cent. of lakes are needed for red tints and from 3 to 8 per cent., together with 10 to 20 per cent. of ochres, for yellow and other shades. The relative concentrations of these materials must be considered when deciding upon the final shade of the rouge.

Some mixtures of mineral powders contain much larger amounts of colour than the everyday toilet powder.

Base for Dry Rouge

	Parts
Osmo-kaolin	16
Zinc stearate	16
Magnesium stearate	10
Zinc oxide	4
Magnesium carbonate	8
Calcium carbonate	46

For pastel or porcelain tints enough titanium oxide is used. (Titanium oxide has three times the whitening power of zinc oxide.)

Base for Fatty Rouge

	Parts
Zinc stearate	30
Magnesium stearate	20
Osmo-kaolin	20
Titanium oxide	6
Calcium carbonate	24

Lakes, ochres and clays are added to give the required colour.

Compact Rouges

Powders such as the above are moistened with a weak solution of gum tragacanth; 1 per cent. dextrin is added to this paste, which is then moulded into compacts in a press.

There is no need to add such materials if the powders contain sufficient kaolin and stearates. Their colour is readily transferred to the puff.

Lip Rouges

Modern lip rouges are improvements of the "grapes" used in the seventeenth century. Such grapes consisted of hard perfumed ointments coloured with black grape juice and orcanet. They (lip rouges) serve the purpose of protecting the mucous membranes of the lips against troubles, and also impart a more or less brilliant and indelible shade.

The origin of lip rouges and their subsequent development were described by the author in *Parfumerie Moderne*, Vol. 30, No. 8, April, 1948—"The Lip Rouges," and it is not proposed to repeat such details here.

Nevertheless, in all seriousness, pride of place must be accorded to the *Cérat Labial* of the French Codex. The recipe represents an official point of view and is given below:

Cérat Labial

	Grammes
White beeswax	50
Petroleum jelly	50
Petroleum oil	2
Rose essence	0·25

It is, as Cerbelaud says (Vol. II, 442), a softening astringent and drying ointment by virtue of its beeswax content, and is very effective against fissures and herpes. To colour this "alcannine" 5 grammes are added. ("Alcannine" is a concentrated extract of orcanet [alkanet] root.)

True cosmetic properties are possessed by vegetable and animal oils, and these oils should be used in preference to petroleum oil. Mixture as

	Grammes
Purified tallow	75
Paraffin	35
Spermaceti	35

is recommended. An alternative is cocoa butter to which beeswax is added.

Such new raw materials have become available during the past few years to manufacturers that considerable advances in lip rouges have been possible. They have made possible the manufacture of sufficiently firm fatty bodies which can readily be moulded and freed from the mould, and which leave a trace of brilliant protective colour on the lips.

Lip cosmetics can be compared with skin preparations from the technical angle. They can be classified into three groups: (*a*) anhydrous fats of the petroleum jelly or lano-petroleum jelly type; (*b*) emulsions with a continuous oil phase—fatty emulsions; and (*c*) emulsions with continuous aqueous phase—vanishing cream type.

The colours used in these products are fat-soluble, or insoluble (pigments) or water-soluble. The rouge is said to be coloured in the mass when fat-soluble colours are used. When the colour is dissolved in the water, the solution is subsequently emulsified.

Rouges Coloured in the Mass

Mainly basic colours are used, together with fatty acids, stearates of rhodamine, chrysoidine, auramine, etc. The resulting colours are not altogether satisfactory even if alcannine (orcanet [alkanet] extract) is used. For quite a time colours soluble in hydrocarbons have been available. Some of these nitro dyes give pleasant scarlet shades, and they can be used to colour petroleum jellies and other fats even when insoluble pigments are used simultaneously with water-soluble colours.

It is absolutely essential for the mineral oil to be "film activated" if the lip preparations are to stick to the mucous membranes. Castor oil, soluble in hydrocarbons, is added to petroleum jellies to achieve this.

Opaque Rouges

Opaque rouges are water-free cosmetics in which the covering power of the highly dispersed opaque lakes is sufficient to mask the imperfections of the mucous membranes. By mixing with titanium oxide, porcelain and pastel shades are obtained. The amount of pigment used can be as much as, or even exceed, 20 per cent. of the total rouge, as the opacity required determines the amount of pigment required. Such rouges can be made from such fats as petroleum jelly, lanolin, cocoa butter, spermaceti, hydrogenated oils. Natural and synthetic waxes can be used as well as oleyl and cetyl alcohols (since 1938), stearates and myristates of glycol, or glycerol and castor oil derivatives. For example:

I

	Parts
White beeswax	31
Paraffin	5
Cocoa butter	7
Cholesterinated petroleum jelly	26
Hydrocarbon-soluble castor oil	4
Benzoinated lard	8
Lakes	19

II

Paraffin oil	21
Petroleum jelly	16
Ceresine	15·5
Paraffin	16·5
Lakes	20

III

	Parts
Hydrogenated castor oil	10
Hydrocarbon-soluble castor oil	17
Cetyl alcohol	7
Beeswax	20
Ozokerite	6
Lanolin	10
Paraffin oil	20
Lakes	10

IV

Beeswax	35
Castor oil	65

V

Beeswax	10
Lanolin	10
Ceresine	37
Paraffin oil	43

Add the required amount of lakes to the formulæ IV and V.

VI

	Grammes
Petroleum jelly	25
Ceresine 64°	25
Paraffin oil	15
Beeswax	15
Lanolin	5
Oleyl alcohol	2
Carnauba wax	3
Lakes	10

Rouges Emulsified in Oily Phase

Emulsion ointments have been known for a long time. Pradal's formula represents their simplest type:

	Grammes
Spermaceti	30
Almond oil	62
Rose milk	2
Powdered tea rose	6

The amount of water—in the Rose Milk—is negligible.

By replacing the petroleum jelly in the formulæ of the preceding section with cholesterinated petroleum jelly approximately 20 per cent of water can be mixed in. The texture of the rouge is not materially altered. Hydrophilic stearic or myristic esters can be incorporated also and they will not affect the final products.

I

	Grammes
White wax	25
Paraffin	10
Cholesterinated petroleum jelly	20
Lanolin	15
Glyceryl ricinoleate	10
Water	20

The fats and waxes are melted and the water, then emulsified with them. Lakes are added and the semi-pasty mixture is moulded. In this way settling of the colour is avoided.

II	Grammes
Paraffin	5
Cetyl alcohol	5
Beeswax	30
Lanolin	15
Monoestol	10
Hydrophilic petroleum jelly	15
Water	20

There is no objection to the use of cold cream formulæ based on beeswax and borax, provided attention is paid to the consistency.

Rouges emulsified in the oily phase can be rendered indelible in one of two ways: (1) By introducing eosine into the fatty acid esters (oleates, stearates, ricinoleates of glycerol or glycol) to the extent of its solubility some 3 to 20 per cent. by weight. (2) By introducing water-soluble dyes into the aqueous phase, such dyes being compatible with the emulsion. Borax emulsions tolerate these additions much better than the cholesterol emulsions. Borax/ cholesterol or borax/ lanolin mixed emulsions are probably the best. Good results are also obtained with hydrophilic petroleum jelly containing octadecyl derivatives of the polyols.

Indelible rouges based on the oily phase are not covered by patents as far as the author is aware. They have a homogeneous, bright appearance, since the fatty phase is visible, and the water phase, because it is dispersed, is invisible. The rouges neither stain the fingers nor seep, and give an excellent colour when applied to the lips. They are readily moulded and remoulded. This type of preparation will become the most popular and will best suit users.

Rouges Emulsified in the Aqueous Phase

Many patents have been taken out by inventors to protect the formulæ which have proved so lucrative. These formulæ are outdated, but it is quite profitable to know the principles on which they are based and the methods of preparation.

These products are hard creams and similar to stearate creams. The emulsifier is a soap, the colour is water-soluble. But the soap, the colour of which is dark, is part of the water phase, and the water forms vacuoles of red or violet dye which can stain the fingers. Rouges based on triethanolamine derivatives as emulsifiers are finer and have a better appearance.

I

	Grammes
Paraffin oil	30
Petroleum jelly	20
Beeswax	10
Stearic acid	6·5
Triethanolamine	1·6
Glycerine or glycol	1
Eosin solution	22·9
Lakes	8
Perfume	2

This rouge is mixed. It gives an opaque shaded coating with an indelible colour underneath it. The colour still persists when every vestige of fat has gone.

II

	Grammes
Beeswax	10
Stearic acid	10
Special triethanolamine stearate	15
Monosteol (ester)	15
Glycol laurate	10
Glyceryl ricinoleate	20
Eosin solution	20

The recipe contains no lakes. About 3 per cent. eosin can be dissolved in the fats and some 20 per cent. in water. The water solubility is increased if glycol is added to the water. It is also possible for some of the eosin to be dispersed throughout the emulsion and not dissolved. The effect of the eosin is at a maximum under these conditions. Yet this type of emulsion never seems to yield the high brilliancy that oil-phase emulsions give.

For the qualities required of a lip-rouge, for the requisite control of its physical properties, for the perfume to employ, for the taste it should have, and for the way it should be used, the reader is referred to the article quoted at the beginning of this chapter.

Powders

Toilet powders are really lightly coloured rouges. They should be as fine as possible. High-speed rotating hammers are used in suitable mills to obtain the requisite fineness. The fine powder is separated by air. Such fine material adheres more readily to the skin. The covering power of the powders varies. Binder has published the following figures (*Chem. and Ind.*, 1924, 555):

Covering Powder

	Parts
Pure titanium oxide	136
Ordinary titanium oxide	81–83
Zinc sulphide	71
Lithopone	52·3
Zinc oxide	50
White lead	31

Titanium oxide reflects 86 per cent. of light, zinc oxide some 77 per cent. and calcium carbonate 60 per cent.

Consideration must be given to the property some substances have of absorbing the skin moisture, while others can absorb the skin fat. Dry skins must be powdered with fatty powders and *vice versa.*

Dry Powder

	Parts
Magnesium carbonate	20
Colloidal kaolin	15
Talcum	20
Lithopone	15
Zinc oxide	25
Titanium oxide	5
Lakes and perfumes	*q.s.*

Semi-fatty Powder

Zinc stearate	20
Magnesium stearate	25
Zinc oxide	15
Titanium oxide	5
Kaolin	10
Calcium carbonate	25
Lakes and perfumes	*q.s.*

Fatty Powder

Zinc stearate	35
Magnesium stearate	15
Zinc oxide	15
Kaolin	10
Calcium carbonate	20

Specialist manufacturers supply lakes in easily adjustable shades, and accordingly it is no longer necessary to use basic compounds in colouring the preparations. It is difficult to follow the fashion in the handbooks.

The powders must be reground with colouring matter and perfume in the Forplex. It must be appreciated that the grinding process can alter the colour, and that particle size also plays a part. Perfumes should be those which have a "powdery" note—*i.e.*, heliotrope, wood essences, methyl ionones and orris products.

Toilet Talcum Powders

As commercial talcum powders are not absolutely white, a small quantity of titanium oxide can be used to correct this fault. Calcium carbonate gives improved adherence and magnesium stearate improved smoothness. Each of these improvements is brought in when baby talcum powders are in process.

	Grammes
Talcum	940
Magnesium stearate	25
Calcium carbonate	25
Titanium oxide	10
Lavender compound	*q.s.*

Beauty Masks

Despite their transient action, masks are frequently used. Sometimes the face is surprisingly rejuvenated by the treatment, and then it is hoped the excellent effect will remain.

It is the manufacturer's object to prepare an unctuous mass which can not only be easily applied in successive layers, but can also be easily removed or cleaned off.

A gelatine mask is the most efficient. When it is applied warm by means of a brush, it will readily set on cooling, and it can then be lifted like a rubber membrane. The behaviour of the mask does not only depend upon the nature of the added materials. It also depends on the *p*H of the gelatine; the iso-electric point of gelatine is lower than that of the skin keratin.

The following is the basic formula:

Gelatine Mask

	Grammes
Powdered or granulated gelatine	40
To be dissolved in:	
Hot water	900
Add:	
Glycerine	30
Titanium or zinc oxide	30

A pink or flesh-tinted lake can be used to colour the preparation. It should only be perfumed with aromatic distilled waters, according to their purpose.

Rose water as astringent.
Orange flower water as hypnotic and sedative.
Lavender water as soothing agent.
Hyssop water as anti-herpes agent.
Garden sage as perspirant.
Cypress and hamamelidis waters as vasomotors.
Camphor or rosemary water as sedative.

Aromatic masks are prepared by adding 400 grammes of the aromatic water to the gelatine dissolved in 500 grammes distilled water. The flower water is added just before the mask is used.

A gum—*e.g.*, gum tragacanth, agar-agar or methyl cellulose—can be used in place of 1 part of the gelatine. The first two suggested alternatives are acid, the third is neutral. Alkaline alginates should be avoided. Glycerinated starch is not excluded. Tapioca arrowroot can be used instead of starch. Glycerine gives it the hydration which is useful in the treatment of dry skins.

II	*Grammes*
Powdered gelatine	25
Hot water	500
Gum tragacanth	20
Glycerinated starch	100
Titanium oxide	15
Distilled floral water	340

The titanium oxide leaves a pearl-like shine on the skin and forms a porcelain-like foundation for further make-up. The gelatine is sometimes replaced by casein, which is also acid. One hundred and fifty grammes casein is required per 1 litre of water. A mixed formula gives good results.

III	*Grammes*
Powdered gelatine	15
Casein	100
Glycerine	25
Zinc oxide	20
Floral water	840

Zinc oxide is amphoteric—*i.e.*, it functions as an acid for alkaline skins and as an alkali in the case of acid skins. So if the skin to be treated is abnormal, zinc oxide is recommended; zones of super-oxidation, acne, scurf, redness, excoriations, and acid or excessively active zones—*e.g.*, shiny nose, yellowish spots in the back—are abnormal.

For the ordinary cases kaolin is more neutral, but artificial bentonite which has been chemically treated and has a *p*H of 10, strongly alkaline, must be avoided. The very acid skins which could withstand such clays are very rare. Their use is very risky, and the effect of contraction of masks does not last.

The absorbent effect of masks is very important. They tend to dry normal skins and still more dry skins (fat-free). This disadvantage can be almost countered by the action of the monoesters of glycerine or glycol emulsified into the gelatinous or clay-containing masses. Moreover, these esters give a satiny effect on the skin and also provide deeply penetrating fatty nourishment.

Fatty Mask

	Grammes
White gelatine	35
Dissolved in:	
Hot water	900
Add:	
Self-emulsifying glycol monoester ..	50
Titanium oxide	15

This can be added to the masks indicated above, whether they contain casein or clays.

Fatty Mask (Almond)

	Grammes
Osmo-kaolin	200
Glycol monomyristate T.G.	50
Hydrophilic almond oil	20
Distilled hot water	400

After emulsification and immediately before use, add:

	Grammes
Laurel or almond water	280

The old preparation based on blanched almonds can be replaced by this mask. For acid masks, containing, *e.g.*, fruit juices, a pure mono-ester emulsified with a small quantity of sulphonated fatty alcohol is used.

Acid, Cleaning Mask

	Grammes
Osmo-kaolin	175
Pure glyceryl monostearate	20
Sulphonated fatty alcohol	5
Water	525
Fruit juice	270

The fruit juice can be expressed from the fruit just before it is used or it can be prepared from a concentrate. It will, of course, be diluted according to its acidity.

Neutral Fatty Mask

	Grammes
Kaolin	120
Oleocetyl alcohol	20
Zinc oxide	40
Lavender water	400
Orange flower water	420

Lecithin can be added to all the formulæ—*e.g.*, in the above the lecithin is taken up in the fatty material and added to the other ingredients immediately before use.

The very astringent masks are useful for flabby, puffy and strained faces, for double chins, etc. Small quantities of the following ingredients may be added to the foregoing formulæ for this purpose: benzoin milk, alum, calamine, zinc carbonate, aluminium acetotartrate, aluminium acetate and tannin. The observations of L. Leduc on masks must be kept in mind. (*Cf.* "Beauty Masks" in *Technique of Beauty Products*, Girardot et Cie, editors 1946, and English Translation, published by Leonard Hill Limited, p. 154.)

As can be understood, the length of time the masks are kept on the face and the conditions of the absorption consequent on their use must be carefully controlled.

Benzoin milk can be prepared to:

	Grammes
Tincture of benzoin (10 per cent.) ..	100
Sulphoricinate *p*H 7	100
Water	800

The milk is easily prepared, it does not curdle and keeps well. Not more than 1 gramme of alum must be used in each mask. Aluminium sulphate is sometimes better tolerated. Such products as the following are inadvisable or even prohibited for masks: mercury and lead salts and radio-active materials. The author does not recommend peroxides, perborates or hydrogen peroxide.

Sometimes thermal muds are effective, but of course only local practitioners who know posology can apply them.

Attention has already been drawn to the fact that the application of the mask can and must be preceded by that of active creams containing organotherapeutic, vitamin, hormone, and carotene substances.

Cream Masks

Cream masks can be marketed for use in the morning, before dressing. They are sufficiently soft for easy dilution and contain active principles.

For preference karaya gum is used, since it does not harden the mixture excessively, and it gives good results.

	Grammes
Karaya gum	40
Glycerine monoester T.G.	88
Titanium or zinc oxide	25
Hydrophilic almond oil	60
Distilled lavender water	785
Antiseptic	2

Glycerinated starch can be added.

Cleansing, acid-reacting cream masks are made by using sulphonated alcohol—a wetting agent—as emulsifier. By adding 1 gramme of salicylic acid to each mask a slight keratolytic effect is obtained. A peeling effect is also obtained. Astringents can be added. Phenaseptate, an antiseptic, has an antitoxic and antipruritic effect on the skin; Peru balsam is both stimulating and healing.

By proper use of these cream masks every morning for a quarter or half an hour before dressing, a marked æsthetic effect is obtained.

4. *LOTIONS*

Face Lotions

There are numerous preparations. The most necessary and the most fashionable are tonic lotions, softening, astringent, vasomotric and acid lotions, but many others can be imagined. Usually they are based on an aromatic distilled water or mixtures of such.

Tonic Alkaline Lotion

	Grammes
Potassium carbonate	1·5
Lauryl sulphonate	3
Glycerine	5
Distilled floral water	90·5

Tonic Neutral Lotion

	Grammes
Tincture of peruvian bark	6
Quillaia tincture	4
Glycerine	5
Rose water	35
Lavender water	50

Softening Lotion

	Grammes
Karaya	3
Boric acid	1
Orthophenyl phenol	1
Clary sage water	20
Lavender water	75

Sulphur Lotion against Acne

	Grammes
Soluble sulphur	1
Camphorated alcohol	1
Artificial rose essence	0·1
Rose water	97·9
Pink colouring *q.s.*	

Dissolve the rose essence in the mixture of camphorated alcohol and soluble sulphur, add the water, and filter.

Astringent Lotion

	Grammes
Alcoholic tannin	0·25
Formaldehyde	0·25
Aromatic water	99·50

Astringent Lotion containing Salicylate

	Grammes
Alcohol 60°	98·5
Menthyl salicylate	0·25
Bornyl salicylate	0·25
Lavender essence	0·25
Artificial jasmine	0·25

Vasomotor Lotion

	Grammes
Witch hazel	40
Cinnamon water	20
Rose water	10
Clove water	30

Acid Lotion

	Grammes
Boric acid	2
Lactic acid	3
Aromatic water	95

Acid Lotion with Strawberry Essence

	Parts
Lactic acid	1
Acetic acid	0·8
Alcoholic strawberry essence (100°)	0·2
Water (distilled from strawberries)	98
Strawberry pink colour *q.s.*	

Eye Lotions

Perfumers are not often asked for eye lotions. So pharmacists could successfully prepare eye specialities, and these could serve well for eye lotions, for are not the eyes one of the main beauty elements of the face?

Distilled waters (eaux) are once again the principal constituents, and it is necessary to consider the distillation of both cornflowers and lime flowers. But these operations can easily be carried out in the laboratory.

For example:

Eye Lotion

	Grammes
Borax	1
Sodium bicarbonate	1
Cornflower water	98

Such a lotion is indispensable in eye-lash make-ups.

A small quantity of sulphonated lauryl alcohol (neutral) can be added so that made-up eyes can be easily cleaned. However, all wetting agents affect the mucosa of the eyes.

Tonic Eye Lotion

	Grammes
Boric acid	5
Borax	2
Glycerine	3
Distilled camphor-water	90

To obtain the last-mentioned water, water is distilled from a mixture of camphor and water.

Corrévon recommends the following plants as suitable for providing rose water for use as eye washes: absinthe, elder, fennel, valerian alone or mixed.

Eyebrow Liquid—To Make Eyebrows and Eyelashes Shiny

	Grammes
Paraffin oil	50
Hydrocarbon-soluble castor oil	48·5
Carotene oil	1
Perfume	0·5

Cosmetic Lotions for the Care of the Skin, according to Aromatherapy Recipes

These lotions are intended for the care of the skin either at home or in beauty establishments. They can be used for aromatising cold or hot water sprays, shower baths, steam baths, frictions or any other lotions which demand the use of aromatic waters or alcohols.

They are usually prepared at 50° or 60° (strength of alcohol). The recipes which follow are for 1 litre.

Tonic Lotion

	Grammes
Terpeneless lavender oil	7
Terpeneless clary sage	3
Tincture of real musk (1 per cent.)	5
Tincture of civet (1 per cent.)	5
Tincture of castoreum (1 per cent.)	5

This is a tonic lotion as well as a sexual balancing agent. When applied to the face it helps to obtain a calm, relieved appearance and can be recommended for strains, overwork, and for application after disturbing nights.

Soothing Lotion

	Grammes
Terpeneless basil oil	3
Essence of clary sage	3
Terpeneless savory oil	1
Terpeneless eau-de-cologne	3

This is a suprarenal tonic lotion and is recommended for exhaustion, continuous tiredness and nervous depression.

Vitalising Carrot Lotion

	Grammes
Terpeneless essence of wild carrot	3
Essence of clary sage	2
Aldehyde complex	5

Carrot derivatives are rightly regarded as giving vigour and vitality to the skin tissues. The aldehyde complexes deserve a certain merit in the same respect.

Sedative Lotion

	Grammes
Essence of neroli water	5
Essence of rose complex	3

A night's sleep is compensated for by this lotion or by orange flower water, a teaspoonful of which is used in the wash-basin and somewhat more in a bath.

Lotion for Underdeveloped Breasts

	Grammes
Terpeneless verbena oil	5
Terpeneless caraway oil	4
Infusion of true musk (1 per cent.) ..	10

It can be used in morning frictions, but is preferably diluted with water. The lotion is intended to firm the breasts and to develop them.

Lotion against Over-development of Breasts

	Grammes
Terpeneless garden sage	3
Terpeneless peppermint oil	2
Terpeneless lavender compound	5

Lotion for Herpes and Eczema

	Grammes
Terpeneless hyssop oil	5
Terpeneless lavender compound	5

Anti-perspirant Lotion

	Grammes
Terpeneless essence of garden sage	5
Eau-de-cologne essence	5

Lotion for Chapped and Cyanotic Hands

	Grammes
Terpeneless rosemary oil	2
Tansy oil	1
Ceylon cinnamon oil	2
Clove oil	1
Artificial carnation (extra)	4

Vasomotor Lotion

	Grammes
Essence of fern compound	5
Terpeneless essence of cypress	2
Crystalline coumarin	3

This lotion has a fine odour of cut grass.

Acne Lotion

	Grammes
Terpineol	8
Artificial lilac	1
Menthyl salicylate	1

Shaving Eczema Lotion

	Grammes
Lavender oil compound	5
Terpeneless menthol	1
Menthyl salicylate	2
Neroli oil	2

Healing Lotion

	Grammis
Soluble Peru balsam	5
Eau-de-cologne essence	5

Lotion for Crusts, Pityriasis, Psoriasis, Seborrhœa, etc.

	Grammes
Moroccan cedar oil	6
Ylang-ylang	1
Lilac compound (extra)	2
Jasmine compound (extra)	1

Friction for Cellulitis

	Grammes
Terpeneless oil of verbena	5
Eau-de-cologne essence	2
Essence of balm mint compound	3

To be dissolved in alcohol diluted with wine vinegar.

Similar lotions can be prepared without alcohol. They are, of course, more dilute. Advantage is taken of the solubilising property of modern wetting agents for the essences. By solubilising them with crystal ricin, translucent lotions similar to Eaux Lustrales are obtained.

The same essences can be used in creams intended for the care of the skin; when this is the case, about 5 grammes of the essential oil complex per kilogramme of the vehicle in the continuous water phase—*e.g.*, cetaline.

Anti-parasite Lotions

Anti-parasite lotions and vinegars have always enjoyed a fairly constant market. To popularise such preparations in the colonial civilisations of the Empire would be a very good thing.

In general these preparations consist of alcoholiç solutions containing essences, oleoresins or synthetics, the anti-parasite activity of which is known.

I

	Grammes
Oleo-resin of pyrethrum	0·2
Essence of artemisia	0·2
Eau-de-cologne essence	0·6
Alcohol 70°	99

II

Oleo-resin of derris	0·2
Chenopodium oil	0·1
Santalol	0·2
Lavender oil	0·5
Alcohol 70°	99

III

Ethyl phthalate	1
Ethyl benzoate	1
Tansy oil	0·2
Rosemary oil	0·2
Artificial rose oil	0·6
Alcohol 75°	97

IV

Oleo-resin of derris	0·2
Benzyl benzoate	1
Thyme oil	0·3
Lavender oil	0·7
Alcohol 60°	97·8

By omitting ethyl phthalate, lustrous lotions or milks are prepared—*e.g.*:

	Grammes
Mixture of essential oils	6
Ricin crystal	4
Water	90

Pyrethrum oleoresin requires a *p*H of 7 or below to exert its activity. Sulpho-ricinates can be obtained buffered to this *p*H. Modern wetting agents, particularly triethanolamine sulphonated lauryl alcohols, can be used to solubilise the products.

Sulphur Lotion for Hair

	Grammes
Dissolved sulphur	20
Karaya solution (2 per cent.)	100
Fatty alcohol sulphonate solution	30
Water	850
Perfume	*q.s.*

Anti-parasite Lotion

	Grammes
Rosemary oil	2
Benzyl benzoate	10
Sodium sulphoricinate	88

Anti-pruritic Lotion

	Grammes
Sylvestran pine oil	3·5
Rosemary oil	2
Garden sage oil	0·5
Moroccan artemisia oil	4
Sulphoricinate (40 per cent.)	90

Healing and Deodorant Lotion

	Grammes
Atlas cedar oil	0·75
Petitgrain oil	1
Lavender oil	2·25
Camphor	4
Sodium sulphoricinate (40 per cent.)	92

The three last lotions must be diluted with water.

Eaux Lustrales

Eaux lustrales are aqueous, strongly perfumed lotions which, while not clear, are not as opaque as milks. As their name indicates, they can be used by women and children in their ablutions. They can also be used in the care of the hair, for fine or ordinary shower baths, for foam douches and for beauty-parlour work.

These preparations can be formulated with a number of ingredients provided sodium sulpho-ricinoleate is used. When, however, crystal ricin is used, the products are more opaque and dissolve greater amounts of essential oils.

Eau Lustrale with Camomile

	Grammes
Camomile perfume compound	1
Ricin crystal	0·5
Water	98·5

Emollient Eau Lustrale

	Grammes
Sulphoricinoleate (50 per cent.) *p*H 7 ..	3
Sodium resorcinate	1
Distilled mallow water	96

Eau Lustrale with Sulphur for Hair

	Grammes
Sulphoricinoleate (50 per cent.)	3
Glyceryl ricinoleate	0·5
Sodium hyposulphite	1
Perfume miscible with castor oil	1
Water	94·5

Anti-alopecia Eau Lustrale

	Grammes
Sodium sulphoricinoleate (50 per cent.) ..	3
Glyceryl ricinoleate	1
Sodium salicylate	0·3
Miscible perfume	0·7
Water	95

Eau Lustrale for Babies

	Grammes
Sulphoricinoleate (50 per cent.)	3
Glyceryl ricinoleate	1
Borax	0·5
Miscible lavender	0·5
Water	95

Methyl cellulose is added to these preparations to increase their viscosity.

Toilet Vinegars

Toilet vinegars have lost some of their former popularity. Despite this they are still necessary and should always be used in those districts of France (and they are numerous) where the well-water has a high calcium content. The latter gradually destroys the acid mantle of the skin, calcifies the epidermis and causes it to wrinkle prematurely. Whereas in the past wine vinegar was used in the preparation of toilet vinegars, today glacial acetic acid or the less penetrating lactic acid is used. Large amounts of acids are unnecessary, as small amounts give solutions with the required low *p*H and are sufficient to neutralise the waters used in washing. Lactic vinegar can be used as an after-shave lotion in order to remove the alkalinity due to soap.

After-shave Vinegar

	Grammes
Lactic acid	0·7
Tincture of benzoin (10 per cent.) ..	2
Eau-de-cologne essence	1
Alcohol 60°	96·3

The alcohol can cause a burning sensation. The amount of essences can be reduced and the alcohol strength reduced to 30°.

For daily use the following is recommended:

Toilet Vinegar

	Grammes
Acetic acid	0·7
Tincture of benzoin (10 per cent.)	2
Lavender compound essence	0·5
Verbena oil	0·5
Alcohol 60°	96·3

Astringent Milk for Enlarged Pores

	Grammes
Acetic acid	0·4
Salicylic acid	0·1
Alum	0·1
Jasmine compound	0·2
Alcohol 40°	99·2

Alcohol-free vinegars are prepared with distilled floral waters.

Alcohol-free Vinegar

	Grammes
Acetic acid	1
Lavender water	30
Clary sage water	29
Rose water	40

A mixture of glycol and butyl glycol can be used to dissolve the synthetic perfumes and terpeneless oils. The toilet vinegar can be strongly perfumed.

Antiseptic Vinegar

	Grammes
Lactic acid	1
Sodium phenaseptate	0·1
Terpeneless lavender oil	0·2
Terpeneless orange oil	0·1
Aldehyde perfume	0·1
Propylene glycol	4
Butyl glycol	4
Water	90·5

Some modern sulphonated fatty alcohols can tolerate a *p*H of about 3·5. Thus it is possible to solubilise the perfumes by mixing them with a suitable wetting agent and thereby obtain a vinegar which not only neutralises the water but softens it. Soaping is thus made easier.

Cleansing Vinegar

	Grammes
Jasmine compound	0·3
Artificial lilac compound	0·3
Eau-de-cologne essence	0·4
Liquid alkyl sulphonate	4
Water	95

Bath Salts

Alkaline salts are usually recommended for these products; neutral salts such as sodium sulphate more rarely so. These products do not soften hard water, and certainly have no beneficial effect on the skin.

Magnesium salts, on the contrary, are regarded as specific products which cause premature ageing. Sulphur derivatives are considered to be capable of restoring elasticity to the skin as well as its resistance to exogenous agents.

Preferably magnesium chloride, magnesium or sodium hyposulphite, magnesium sulphate may be recommended. Most of these salts are supplied in transparent crystals. Although magnesium chloride is hygroscopic, it is less so if mixed with the sulphate in sufficient quantity.

The crystals are mixed off with the perfume in a coating pan.

Sulphur Salts

	Parts
Sodium hyposulphite	99
Perfume	1

Magnesium Salts

	Parts
Magnesium hyposulphite	33
Magnesium sulphate	33
Magnesium chloride	33
Perfume	1

Oxidising Reducing Salts

	Parts
Sodium hyposulphite	96
Manganese chloride	3
Iron sulphate	0·2
Perfume	0·8

Reducing Salts

	Parts
Sodium hyposulphite	98·5
Potassium iodide	0·5
Perfume	1

5. *DENTIFRICES*

Toothpastes

Because of war conditions (1939-45) it became necessary to give up glycerites of starch for use in toothpastes. These well-known vehicles took up large quantities of calcium carbonate in an able manner. Calcium carbonate is the abrasive generally used for the cleaning of teeth.

Present-day dentifrices usually dry up at the tube orifice, as they contain little or no glycerine; sorbitol syrups, glycol and its derivatives are usually unsuitable substitutes for glycerine.

Dentifrice with Starch

	Parts
Glycerite of starch	30
Glycerine	25
Water	15
Precipitated calcium carbonate	30
Carmine naccarat *q.s.*	
Mint flavour *q.s.*	

English Formula

	Parts
Glycerite of starch	12
Glycerine	11·5
Milk of magnesia	22
Magnesium carbonate	12
Calcium carbonate	16
Petroleum oil	1·5
Saccharine	0·1
Barley flour	5
Water	19·9
Antiseptic *q.s.*	
Perfume *q.s.*	

Nowadays gum gels replace the glycerite of starch—*e.g.*, those of gum tragacanth, alginic acid or its salts, and methyl cellulose. The last mentioned is inert to the effect of the calcium ion and does not deteriorate on keeping. Saccharine is used to give sweetness to the paste and geranium or cyclamen lake for the colour—*e.g.*:

Methyl Cellulose Dentifrice

Methyl cellulose gel	65 parts
Precipitated calcium carbonate	34 ,,
Rose lake	1 ,,
Saccharine	1 gramme
Perfume *q.s.*	

Warm water is placed in a mixing tank. The gum is added and left to swell for 24 hours before it is used. The remaining ingredients are added and mixed in until the mixture is homogeneous.

Bentonite is no longer used as a gelling agent as it gives unsatisfactory results.

The calcium carbonate must be free from associated minerals, and neutral. As its *p*H is relatively high it can attack aluminium tubes and cause them to swell. Soap, which is added to toothpaste as a foaming agent, can cause similar effects. It is therefore highly desirable to buffer the calcium carbonate either with dicalcium phosphate or with magnesium carbonate. Soap is replaced by a tasteless sulphonated fatty alcohol chosen from those with a *p*H of 7.

The following is another recipe:

	Grammes
Gum mucilage	50
Calcium carbonate	30
Magnesium carbonate	7
Sulphonated fatty alcohol	3
Sweetening agent, perfume and colour *q.s.*	

Some makers prefer alkaline toothpastes which they fill into tin or tin-coated lead tubes. Such pastes neutralise the acidity of thrush as well as that of "dental film" of the teeth. Borax, 2 to 3 per cent., and soap powder are equally effective. Hitherto, soaps made from almond oil or cocoa butter have been used, but today, when customers are much more exacting, fine-lather soaps are preferred to coconut/palm kernel soaps. Other makers use sodium sulphoricinoleate or other non-lathering detergents or emulsions based on self-emulsifying glycol myristate.

Dark red dentifrice pastes are coloured with eosine, rhodamine or carmine S.S. The amount used depends on the tint and intensity required.

The flavour is usually based on essences of mint, menthol and anise,* and the composition contains such antiseptic phenols as clove or thyme. Cinnamon is liked, and the strongly flavoured tarragon can be added to it. Caraway, cumin, coriander and fennel are also used. Although American chewing gums have popularised chewing-gum flavours, they have not justified the use of methyl salicylate. It is thus necessary to replace curled mint oils by those of peppermints.

The essence of Rambiasana of Madagascar is regarded as having very suitable properties for such dental troubles as gingivitis.

* See perfumes for dentifrices, pp. 51, 52, 53.

Since it has an aroma of rose, it can be used to replace the very much more expensive rose essence.

Other active products such as rhatany extract, catechu, Para cress, pyrethrum, cinchona and quillaia are added to dentifrices, pastes, powders and solutions. Phenols, salols, mercury salts, perborates and fluorides should be avoided.

Dentifrice Powders

Dentifrice powders do not have an attractive appearance. They should be sold in cartons provided with a brush-shaped orifice, which can be closed by means of a screw, so that the powder is not spilled during use. Perborate powders are far too alkaline, and are accordingly buffered with dicalcium phosphate. Most if not all modern powders contain a lathering agent.

I

	Grammes
Precipitated calcium carbonate	70
Soap powder	5
Borax	5
Magnesium carbonate	18
Rose lake and perfume	2

II

Precipitated calcium carbonate	60
Magnesium carbonate	25
Di-calcium phosphate	5

It is easy to prepare finely divided powders which are pleasant to use and are reasonable in price on such a basis.

No hard abrasives are used in these preparations. It is very desirable not to use powdered pumice, dry bone, coral, even kaolin, which sometimes contains silica grains, or such powdered products as orris, licorice and pyrethrum, which tend to wet the powder containing them and to ferment.

Elixirs and Dentifrice Waters

Dentifrice waters and elixirs consist of alcoholic solutions of essential oil complexes (*e.g.*, mint, anise, cinnamon, clove, thyme, tarragon, etc.), with or without sialogogic products (*e.g.*, essence of garden sage or tonics and astringents—*e.g.*, rhatany extract, cinchona, etc.).

They are used for rinses and mouthwashes after cleaning with pastes or powders.

I

	Parts
Alcohol	98·7
Dentifrice essence	1
10 per cent. tincture of benzoin	0·1
Oleo-resin of vanilla	0·2
Liquid red colouring	*q.s.*

There is a strong tendency for these products to be replaced by aqueous solutions of essential oils solubilised by strong wetting agents such as the triethanolamine or ammonia sulphonated alcohols.

For example:

II

	Parts
Solubilising wetting agent	10
Dentifrice essence	2
Water	88
Colour	*q.s.*

These solutions are used in place of the former liquid dentifrice potassium coconut soaps.

III

	Parts
Liquid coconut soap (18 per cent.)	98
Dentifrice essence	2
Colour	*q.s.*

These soaps, although clear in summer temperatures, become turbid at low temperatures because of the high melting point of the higher fatty acid soaps. The fault can be eliminated if alcohol is added to the soaps.

IV

	Parts
Liquid coconut soap (18 per cent.)	58
Alcohol 95°	40
Dentifrice essence	2
Red colour	*q.s.*

V

Liquid coconut soap	54
Alcoholate of pyrethrum roots	2
Tincture of para cress	2
Dentifrice essence	2
Alcohol 90°	40
Colour	*q.s.*

The monograph on "Dentifrices" in *Parfumerie Moderne* should be read.

6. *HAIR PRODUCTS*

Light Separable Brilliantines

Separable brilliantines consist of two layers, the lower one an alcoholic or aqueous solution of alcoholic or water-soluble products, the upper one a solution of essential oil and fatty products in a hydrocarbon of the deodorised kerosene type. Into such products there is a tendency to introduce active products—*e.g.*, castor oil soluble in hydrocarbons.

Care must be taken to avoid dissolving in the water partially fat-soluble materials and in the hydrocarbon hydrophilic products. By taking this precaution contamination of the interface between the layers is avoided. Calcium salts in the water can give insoluble opaque fatty acid soaps of calcium. This is the reason for the preferred use of a double-distilled or electrolytically purified water.

Simple Separable Brilliantine

	Grammes
Kerosene	3
Bergamot oil	1
Orange oil	1
Alcohol 25°	95
Chlorophyll	*q.s.*

Light Separable Brilliantine Containing Sulphur

	Grammes
Castor oil soluble in hydrocarbons	1
Kerosene	2
Lavender oil	1
Orange oil	1
Sodium hyposulphite solution (2 per cent.)	95
Yellow dye	*q.s.*

Antiseptic Fatty Light Separable Brilliantine

	Grammes
Kerosene	2
Oleyl alcohol	1
Lemon oil	1
Tangerine oil	1
Hydroxyquinoline	0·1
Water	94·9

Antiseptic Light Separable Brilliantine

	Grammes
Kerosene	1
Castor oil soluble in hydrocarbons	1
Bergamot oil	2
Water	96·5
Formaldehyde (40 per cent.)	0·5

Light Separable Brilliantine with Pantothenic Acid

	Grammes
Kerosene	3
Bergamot compound oil	2
Soluble castor oil	0·5
Pantothenic acid	0·5
Water	94

An alcoholic solution of B_2 vitamin or a para-amino benzoic acid solution of similar concentration can replace pantothenic acid, which is not generally available.

Brilliantines and Hair Oils with Film-forming Properties

People who lived in times earlier than our own used to anoint their hair with fatty substances. Nowadays, it seems that dry hair is preferred. Vegetable oils make for dark and dull hair because the natural fats penetrate into the hair fibres and make them more transparent. Mineral oils, on the other hand, have no affinity for the hair and do not really grease it, but they do remain at the surface. But it is difficult to render mineral oils soluble. This, in turn, leads to stronger and yet more powerful shampoos which leave the hair dry and free of sebum. The excessive treatment the hair has to undergo and the almost daily use of strong detergents lend a great interest to modern hair preparations with a surface-active effect, particularly to those which can nourish the hair without making it dull.

So-called brilliantines should give the hair a special lustre. Such a lustre requires a microscopically thin layer of the brilliantine—*i.e.*, the layer must be only a few Ångströms thick. Thus the oil must have a high spreading power, must be liquid and unctuous, and must be prepared according to the scientific principles of surface physics. Explanations of such phenomena have already been given and will not be repeated here. (*Cf. Traitements Capillaires P.M.*, 39, December, 1946.) By adding a polarised oil capable of being oriented while adhering to the hair, the mineral oils can be made both film-forming and unctuous.

I	*Parts*
Petroleum oil (0·880)	95
Castor oil soluble in hydrocarbons ..	5

Dyes directly soluble in the oil are used to colour the preparation. Perfuming is carried out with perfumes the solubility of which is greater in oil than in alcohol.

Mixture I above is too viscous to be applied by means of a spray, but it can be made more liquid with a low density odourless kerosene or with the liquid, adherent oleyl ester, or even with both these materials. Liquid petroleum oils with a density of 0·875 or 0·865 can now be obtained.

II

	Grammes
Paraffin oil	75
Oleyl ester	10
Deodorised kerosene	10
Soluble castor oil	5

The quantity of castor oil in these products can be increased because of the low viscosity of both the diluents and oils.

III

	Grammes
Light petroleum oil (0·865)	79
Soluble castor oil	20
Perfume and colouring	1

The brilliantines based on petroleum products are not the only products which provide suitable lustre and nourishment to the hair. Chemists have evolved super-glycerinated or glycolated oils which nourish the hair and yet neither dull it nor impair and prevent the waving. These oils do not readily become rancid. They can be supplemented with fat-soluble vitamins or provitamin A, so as to replace the natural vitamin-containing oils—*e.g.*, avocado oil. According to their origin, the oils are termed almond-sebum, corn-sebum and groundnut-sebum. Small quantities of lecithin, vitamin F or its glycol derivative can be dissolved in the oils with the advantage that they make combing easier.

Oleic acid monoesters, whatever their source, are soluble in alcohol, and this allows homogeneous alcohol brilliantine to be prepared. The dilution of the oil renders it very easy to spread the oil in a thin, easily absorbable layer.

	Grammes
Alcohol 93°	50
Liquid monoester	48
Perfume and colouring	*q.s.*

Such brilliantines appear to be much more preferable than those based on two phases (separable type) in which petroleum oils were used in place of vegetable oils so as to avoid the formation of a slimy layer at the interface. These two layer products are not of much interest as brilliantines, yet when the new oils are used the brilliantines containing them nourish the hair without making it greasy, their diluted solutions remain clear and homogeneous, and they do not become rancid. Moreover, the minimum quantity of alcohol necessary to make them sprayable need be used.

	Grammes
Groundnut monoester	70
Alcohol 95°	29
Lecithin, glycolated vitamin, perfume and colouring	1

Solidified Brilliantines

The technique for the preparation of so-called brilliantines crystallisé may also be modified. Hitherto such preparations have been of the petroleum jelly type, already studied, to which wax or spermaceti was added.

I

	Grammes
Petroleum jelly	40
Paraffin oil	40
Spermaceti	2
White wax (beeswax)	2
Ceresine	2
Paraffin	2

These materials are difficult to remove from the hair even with powerful shampoos, and they cause their lather to collapse. To improve their spreading properties, hydrocarbon-soluble castor oil is added to them. Spreading with the brush is made much easier. Cholesterol can also be added so as to provide nourishment and at the same time facilitate cleansing.

II

	Grammes
Pure petroleum jelly	40
Artificial petroleum jelly	49
Cholesterol	1
Soluble castor oil	1

By using solid derivatives of castor oil monoesters much less greasy solid brilliantines can be made which have the added advantages of not dulling the hair and being easily removed.

	Grammes
Monoricinoleate	70
Cetyl alcohol	30
Perfume	*q.s.*

These brilliantines are very shiny, very fatty, and yet are easily removed by washing and facilitate both combing and brushing.

Brilliantine Emulsions

Brilliantines are now made in the form of semi-liquid, very bright, shiny creams.

I	Grammes
Hydrophilic petroleum jelly	20
Petroleum oil	20
Water	60

Melt the fats at 40°. Add the water, mix vigorously and homogenise.

II	Grammes
Hydrophilic petroleum jelly	10
Petroleum oil	30
Water	60
Antiseptic and perfume	*q.s.*

These emulsions are made into fixative brilliantines by the addition of a gum solution—*e.g.*, 2 per cent. gum karaya.

Hair Fixatives

The so-called fixatives are in fact gum mucilages.

I	Grammes
Gum tragacanth	4
Water	95
Antiseptic	1
Colouring and perfume	*q.s.*

Contrary to what has earlier been said, fixatives can be changed to brilliantines by adding fatty materials to them. Castor oil could only be employed with difficulty with gums hitherto, but now super-glycolated castor oils form stable emulsions with gums.

II	Grammes
Gum tragacanth gel	93
Crystalline castor oil with 30 per cent. free oil	5
Glycol mono-ricinoleate	2

III	
Gum gel	90
Hydrophilic petroleum jelly	10

If the gum tragacanth is replaced by gum karaya the fixatives are liquids.

While calcium alginate has been recommended for gum-containing preparations in paste form, it has the disadvantage that it forms films on the hair as it dries and is therefore of little interest. Methyl cellulose has the same disadvantage, but not quite to the same extent.

IV	Grammes
Methyl cellulose	4
Water	96
Perfume, antiseptic and colour	*q.s.*

The mucilage may be emulsified with hydrophilic oils as above.

Hair Creams with Film-forming Properties

The capillary or film-forming technique for applying cream to the hair after it has been permanently waved so as to restore part of the fats removed from the hair by the alkaline treatment is becoming more and more popular. Glycol and glycerol mono-myristates are preferably used, and they yield semi-liquid emulsions. By virtue of the low melting point of the fatty acid, the emulsions penetrate deeper into the hair.

I	Grammes
Glycol monomyristate T.G. self-emulsifying	16
Hydrophilic oil (amygdaline)	8
Glycol mono-ricinoleate	6
Water	70
Antiseptic	*q.s.*

II	
Cétasal	20
Paraffin oil	6
Vegetable oils	16
Lecithin	3
Glyceryl ricinoleate	5
Water	50
Antiseptic	*q.s.*

Vitamin F or preferably its ester may also be used. When lecithin is used the quantity of antiseptic must be increased.

A similar emulsion is obtained if about 10 per cent. of sulphonated cetyl alcohol is used.

Hair Creams containing Marrow and having Film-forming Properties

Marrow is used because it has specific properties. The unctuous phosphorus-containing fat gives a special brilliancy to the hair and penetrates the hair fibres without dulling them. In addition, it facilitates combing of the hair and does not spoil the curls.

It is produced either as a glycol or petroleum extract. They are products obtained after a methodical extraction with solvents which differ according to the use to which it is intended to put them. They are used in shampoos or in creams having film-forming properties. The amount of preservative must of necessity be increased.

	Grammes
Film-forming cream	95–98
Marrow extract	5–2

This is a typical preparation:

	Parts
Glycol stearate T.G. (self-emulsifiable)	11
Glycerol stearate T.G.	2
Water	75
Antiseptic	0·3

Heat while stirring. Furthermore, melt

	Parts
Soya lecithin	2

in

Hydrophilol (hydrophilic oil)	9·4
Perfume	0·3

Pour this mixture into the former and stir until it is cool. The cream is soft (hardness approximately between 10 and 30). A petroleum extract of marrow is added to the cream prepared as described.

Shampoos

Shampoos are essentially liquid soaps consisting of the potassium soaps of coconut oil and palm-kernel oil. The soaps have no free alkali, yield an abundant lather and clean the hair well. Solubilised essential oil complexes are used for perfume as they dissolve directly in the dilute soap. Here is an example:

Juniper Shampoo

Liquid soap with 18 per cent. fatty acid	1 litre
Miscible juniper perfume	5 grammes
Brown colour	*q.s.*

Occasionally the content of fatty acids is reduced to 12 per cent., but as the soap is now too liquid, it is thickened with a mucilage.

Camomile Shampoo

	C.c.
Liquid soap (12 per cent.)	800
Stipine solution (10 per cent.)	200
Miscible camomile perfume	5
Golden-yellow colour	*q.s.*

Stipine is a sodium alginate paste. About one-tenth of dry or very pure alginate can be used.

Triethanolamine stearate gives a finer lather than coconut oil. It can also be used:

Shampoo with Triethanolamine Soap

	C.c.
Liquid soap (12 per cent.)	950
Triethanolamine oleate	50
Perfume and colouring	*q.s.*

Super-fatted shampoos containing free oil are obtained by utilising the properties of crystalline castor oil—*e.g.*, castor oil soap containing 20 to 30 per cent. unsaponified oil. Thus 2 to 5 per cent. free castor oil can be introduced without causing turbidity in the shampoo. The shampoo becomes very unctuous and lends brilliancy to the hair and does not dull it.

Shampoo with Castor Oil

	C.c.
Liquid soap (12 per cent.)	900
Castor oil (crystal type)	100
Perfume and colouring	*q.s.*

Lecithin, dissolved in cetyl alcohol, is found in the so-called "egg-shampoos." While the lecithin makes hair combing easier, the cetyl alcohol imparts gloss.

Egg Shampoo

	C.c.
Liquid soap (12 per cent.)	900
Castor oil (crystal type)	90
Oleo-cetyl alcohol	8
Lecithin	2
Perfume and yellow colour	*q.s.*

Non-lathering oil shampoos have lost their former popularity. They are sodium sulpho-ricinoleate solutions.

Non-foaming Shampoo

	Grammes
Sulphoricinoleate (50 per cent.)	200
Stipine solution (10 per cent.)	100
Water	700
Perfume and colour	*q.s.*

These shampoos may be superfatted or lecithin may be added as before.

For several years now preference has been shown for sulphonated fatty alcohols neutralised with soda, potash, ammonia or triethanolamine. Numerous other synthetics have been developed —*e.g.*, sulphonates of polyvalent alcohol esters, sulphonates of amino-alcohol amides and alkyl aryl sulphonates. The sodium salts, in paste and powder forms, are not very soluble in water (or at least give turbid solutions which have to be clarified with glycols and glycol esters, benzyl alcohol, etc.). They often contain residual sodium sulphate. The ammonia and triethanolamine salts are semi-liquid and yield clear solutions.

These shampoos, because of their strong detergent properties, have the drawbacks of drying the hair and making it frizzy as well as stripping it of its essential lipids. Since the solutions are too thin they are thickened with stipine (sodium alginate) solutions. Methyl cellulose mucilages coagulate in the presence of soaps. Because they are often acid they have to be buffered with small amounts of caustic potash or ammonia in order to bring their *p*H to about 6 to 7. Below this *p*H they decompose the potassium soap and castor oil, if used.

Fatty Alcohol Shampoo

	Grammes
Fatty alcohol sulphonate (ammoniacal 30 per cent.)	100
Caustic potash (approximately)	3
Castor oil (crystal type)	37
Water	760
Colour and perfume	*q.s.*

The sulphonated alcohols can tolerate large amounts of castor oil soap without losing their power of lathering. Their emollient effect is increased, and they give the hair a perfect gloss and at the same time nourish the hair by means of the oil penetrating into the shafts.

Fatty Alcohol Shampoo with Castor Oil

	Grammes
Sulphonated fatty alcohol (30 per cent.)	120
Castor oil (crystal type)	100
Water	780
Perfume and colour	*q.s.*

These solutions, coupled with the so-called egg shampoos, give very good results.

Fatty Alcohol Shampoo with Eggs

	Grammes
Sulphonated fatty alcohol (20 per cent.) ..	120
Crystalline castor oil	60
Cetyl alcohol	8
Egg lecithin	2
Water	810
Yellow colour and perfume	*q.s.*

Marrow-fat extracts are added to shampoos because they provide excellent nourishment for the hair and do not dull it.

Clear Shampoo with Marrow

	C.c.
Fatty alcohol shampoo	980
Glycol extract of marrow	20
Perfume and colour	*q.s.*

Often, however, cloudy or milky shampoos are preferred.

Milky Shampoo with Marrow

	C.c.
Fatty alcohol shampoo	970
Petroleum extract of marrow	30
Perfume and colour	*q.s.*

A hydrophilic oil may also be added to give a more or less opaque shampoo.

Milky Shampoo with Oil

	C.c.
Fatty alcohol shampoo	980
Hydrophilic groundnut oil	20
Perfume and colour	*q.s.*

Opaque Shampoo with Castor Oil

	C.c.
Fatty alcohol shampoo	970
Glyceryl ricinoleate	30
Perfume and colour	*q.s.*

Saponin, which is often recommended as an addition to shampoos, is unnecessary since it does not increase the lather.

Shampoo with Sulphur

	C.c.
Fatty alcohol shampoo	990
Dissolved sulphur	10

This addition may appear to have no effect because of the rapid action of the shampoo, but the sulphur combines with the hair keratin and makes it more elastic and more suitable for waving. Juniper-scented sulpho-compounds are used, as has already been mentioned. Another useful addition is vitamin F in the form of glycol isolinoleate.

Vitaminised Shampoo

	C.c.
Fatty alcohol shampoo	980
Hydrophilic vitamin F	20

As some 30 per cent. fatty alcohol and castor oil shampoos are normally gels they can be filled into tin-coated lead tubes.

Shampoo for Tubes

	C.c.
Triethanolamine sulphated fatty alcohol (30 per cent.)	850
Castor oil	150
Perfume	*q.s.*

Lastly, the normal type of good shampoo preparations, especially the mixed sort. They have good lathering and detergent properties, are harmless to the hair yet efficient in their effect, and but slightly acid, even if unctuous.

Mixed Shampoo

	C.c.
Liquid soap	500
Triethanolamine lauryl sulphonate ..	50
Water	450
Perfume and colour	*q.s.*

Most of the foregoing formulæ can be combined one with the other. Thus it is possible to develop a wide range of products suitable for different uses.

Sulphur and Juniper Shampoo

	Grammes
Sulphonated fatty alcohol (6 per cent. solution)	99
Sulphur sulpho-conjugated cedria	1

PERMANENT-WAVE SOLUTIONS

Cold permanent waving is the only process that demands, at present, numerous different special preparations. It is said that the keratine of the hair is altered when the hair is heated in the presence of alkalies. The altered keratine retains the new form imparted to it during its chemical modification.

Ammonia solution was first used to produce waves on curlers. The action of the ammonia is rapid and almost harmless, as it quickly vaporises and reduces the temperature of the heating apparatus.

Ammoniacal Solution

	Grammes
Volatile alkali (21 per cent.)	300–400
Water	700–600

Borax strengthens the hair and is accordingly used:

Ammoniacal Borax Solution

	Grammes
Ammonia	140–300
Borax	40–10
Water	820–690

As can be imagined, the smell of ammonia rapidly becomes unbearable in hairdressing saloons, and accordingly non-volatile alkalies were used to overcome this trouble. Sodium, potassium or ammonium carbonate were used.

Ammonia-free Solution

	Grammes
Sodium or potassium carbonate	100
Water	900

Ammonia-free Borax Solution

	Grammes
Sodium or potassium carbonate	180
Borax	20
Water	800

It will be seen that widely differing amounts of ingredients are used. Different types of hair do not react in the same way; blond is very sensitive, auburn hair less so, and black hair is highly resistant. There is therefore ample reason to increase gradually the solution strength, having regard to the time the heat is applied and to the firmness of the treated hair.

The bleached hair is very brittle. Oxidation usually destroys the surface keratine of such hair, which has a fine texture and still contains, on occasion, traces of oxygen. Hence a reducing agent such as sodium or potassium sulphite is added to the solution.

Solution for Bleached Hair

	Grammes
Sodium carbonate	80
Borax	10
Sodium sulphite	20
Water	890

It is very desirable to carry out preliminary tests on a part of the hair to be treated to determine the best concentration and most suitable processing time.

Solution for Brittle Hair

	C.c.
Ammonia 21°	200
Sodium carbonate	40
Sodium or potassium sulphite	20
Water	740

Triethanolamine may be used.

Solution Formula after Navarre

	Grammes
Ammonium carbonate	40
Potassium sulphite	20
Borax	30
Triethanolamine	120
Water	790

Solution I (Soap, Perfumery and Cosmetics) *(after Ralph Auch)*

	Grammes
Sodium carbonate	4·5
Ammonium carbonate	2·5
Borax	26·5
Potassium sulphite	55
Water, sufficient to	1,000

Solution II *(after Ralph Auch)*

	Grammes
Potassium carbonate	55
Borax	26·5
Sodium carbonate	4·5
Ammonium carbonate	2·5
Water, sufficient to	1,000
Perfume	*q.s.*

Frequently shampooed hair is woolly because it does not contain its original fatty components. Fatty acids are accordingly added to permanent-waving solutions.

Fatty Solution

Alkaline solution	1 litre
Sodium sulphoricinoleate	10–60 grammes

This solution remains clear. Today there is a tendency to use cloudy, translucent or milky solutions.

Milky Solution

	C.c.
Alkaline solution	950
Sodium sulphoricinoleate	40
Hydrophilol (hydrophilic oil)	10

These quantities can be considerably increased.

Cerbelaud gives the following:

Fatty Solution

	Grammes
Sodium sulphite	90
Sodium carbonate	90
Water	820

Immediately before use is added:

Castor oil	120 grammes

If a homogeneous solution is preferred:

Fatty Solution

	C.c.
Alkaline solution	900
Sulphoricinoleate	70
Glycol ricinoleate	30

The use of triethanolamine oleate is also recommended.

Fatty Solution with Triethanolamine Oleate

	C.c.
Alkaline solution	900
Triethanolamine oleate	100

Some fatty alcohols impart gloss. To disperse them ammonium or triethanolamine lauryl sulphonate is used.

Solution with Fatty Alcohols

	C.c.
Alkaline solution	900
Ammonium lauryl sulphonate	70
Oleo-cetyl alcohol	30

Either oleyl or cetyl alcohol may be used. Lastly, there are alcohols from wool wax. They are viscous, very shiny and can be solubilised.

Solution with Lanolin

	C.c.
Alkaline solution	900
Ammonium lauryl sulphonate (30 per cent.)	70
Wool alcohol	30

The amounts can be varied according to the results intended. Marrow extracts, which are more active, can be used.

The patents quoted by Morelle in *Traitements Capillaires*, p. 14, are:

U.S.P. 2,095,374

	Grammes
Potassium sulphite	200
Potassium carbonate	430
Ammonium sulphite	360

To be dissolved according to requirements.

British Patent—Knibbs

	Grammes
Mono-ethanolamine sulphite	80
Mono-ethanolamine	60
Cyclohexanol	10

for 1 litre.

French Patent 813,334

	Grammes
Lanolin	25
Sodium carbonate	5
Sodium sulphite	20
Ammonia	20
Ammonium sulpho-ricinoleate	25

for 1 litre.

Ammonium thioglycollate solutions, 5 to 8 per cent. acid, are used for cold permanent waves. The solutions help the formation of new sulphur bridges in the hair keratin and no heat need be used. The product is supplied together with an oxidising rinse. A lukewarm permanent wave is carried out with a solution of half the strength, about 4 per cent. acid (maximum strength). The solution is applied without raising the temperature to boiling.

Solution for Cold Wave

	Grammes
Thioglycollic acid	51
Ammonia 0·880	43
Water to	1,000

Strong Solution II

	Grammes
Thioglycollic acid	63
Ammonia 0·880	54
Water to	1,000

Depilatories

Depilatory powders, to be diluted with water immediately before use, are generally based on barium sulphide, sometimes with neutral products or analgesics. The sulphides are such powerful solvents for keratin that their action must be limited to the hair, and they must not attack the skin. All sulphides do not have the same action. Once a specific compound has been adopted it is advisable to use it to the exclusion of others. Consistent results can then be obtained.

Depilatory Powder

	Grammes
Barium sulphide	35
Titanium oxide	25
Starch	39·8
Powdered menthol	0·2

Zinc oxide tends to limit the alkaline reaction and soap favours the washing.

Depilatory Powder with Zinc Oxide

	Grammes
Barium sulphide	25
Soap powder	5
Starch	40
Zinc oxide	30

Francis Chilson recommends benzocaine 0·2 per cent. as the analgesic. Strontium sulphide is sometimes used instead of barium sulphide.

Depilatory Agent with Strontium Sulphide

	Grammes
Strontium sulphide	35
Starch	35
Talcum	29·8
Menthol or benzocaine	0·2

Mixed Depilatory Agent

	Grammes
Strontium sulphide	25
Barium sulphide	10
Starch	20
Calcium carbonate	45

Perfumes are almost always altered by the depilatory preparations. Wood essences, particularly cedar oil, are much more resistant.

Phyllis Jacobs

Depilatory pastes are usually suspensions of these powders in gum solutions. They often solidify and become useless in the presence of calcium carbonate or zinc oxide.

Depilatory Paste

	Grammes
Strontium sulphide	15
Barium sulphide	15
Glycerinated starch	68
Wood perfume	2

Epilating Waxes

Epilating waxes are of the resinous pitch type. They are softened immediately before use by soaking them in warm water. They mat the hair in the area to which they are applied, and when the cold wax is pulled away it takes the matted hair with it.

Epilating Wax I

	Grammes
Light resin or colophony	50
Yellow beeswax	25
Paraffin	20
Petroleum jelly	5

Epilating Wax II

	Grammes
Colophony	40
Wax or resin	38
Carnauba wax	6
Petroleum oil	15
Perfume	1

7. *NAIL PREPARATIONS*

Nail Polishes

Nail polishes are in very great demand. They can be simply prepared by dissolving cinema film stripped of its gelatine by a wash in boiling water acidified with hydrochloric acid. A mixture of acetone and amyl acetate is most often used as the solvent. The polish obtained from film celluloid is flexible because the film was plasticised with camphor.

Colourless Polish

I

	Parts
White celluloid	8
Amyl acetate	22
Acetone	70

If cellulose nitrate is available the formula becomes:

II

	Parts
Cellulose nitrate	5
Amyl acetate	25
Acetone	70

Cellulose nitrate or gun-cotton is generally supplied as a 40 per cent. collodion solution in butyl alcohol. With other solvents the earlier formula becomes:

III

Collodion (40 per cent.)	20 parts
Butyl acetate	20 grammes
Ethyl acetate	40 ,,
Propyl acetate	20 ,,

For greater gloss and hardness some makers recommend the addition of such resins as benzoin and sandarac. More plasticiser is necessary when camphor-free collodion and resins are used, and such materials as butyl tartrate, ethyl phthalate and even castor oil. The nail polish is rendered sticky and slow drying when an excess of the last mentioned is used. Tricresyl phosphate is sometimes employed.

Plasticised Varnish

	Parts
Varnish No. III	95
Ethyl phthalate	5

Various other solvents can be used in addition to those already mentioned—*e.g.*, ethyl lactate, methyl acetate, methyl ethyl ketone, di-acetone alcohol, ethyl and methyl propionates, mesityl oxide, propyl, isopropyl, butyl and amyl alcohols.

Nail varnishes of the transparent type are coloured with organic solvent-soluble colours. A standard solution of the colour is prepared and tests are carried out in order to ascertain the required amounts necessary. Lacquer varnishes are obtained by mixing a rapidly drying cellulose paint of the desired shade with one of the above-mentioned polishes. Mixtures of paints of the same type of products, Duc Ripolin, can also be used.

Lacquer Varnish

	Parts
Colourless nail polish	70
Lacquer paint	20
Solvent mixture	10

The solvent must be chosen so as to be suitable for the paint. A homogeneous product will then be obtained.

Nail Polish Solvents

Solvents for nail polishes are sold as specialty lines, and usually consist of mixtures of the solvents indicated above—*e.g.*:

Acetone Solvent

	Parts
Butyl acetate	20
Ethyl acetate	20
Acetone	40
Amyl acetate	20

Because both acetone and amyl acetate have unpleasant odours they need not be used.

Acetone-free Solvent

	Parts
Butyl acetate	20
Ethyl acetate	40
Propyl alcohol	40

French users of nail polishes do not like solvents such as toluene, benzene or naphtha, which are used in other countries, for their polishes or solvents.

Fatty Solvent

	Parts
Butyl acetate	35
Ethyl acetate	60
Soluble castor oil	5

The castor oil can be replaced by vitamin F.

Strong Remover

	Parts
Ethyl acetate	50
Butyl ethylene glycol	20
Acetone	30

Methyl ethylene glycol and butyl stearate can be used in nail-polish removers. Oleyl acetate can be employed to obtain a fatty effect.

Nail Polishing Powders

Nail-polishing powders are mainly based on the fine polishing producing tin oxide. Other substances such as kaolin, titanium oxide, zinc stearate are used with it.

Nail-polishing Powder

	Parts
Tin oxide	60
Zinc stearate	20
Titanium oxide	20

The powder can be coloured pink with a suitable lake.

Kieselguhr or siliceous diatomite powder is an excellent polisher, somewhat more powerful than the ones given earlier and certainly cheaper.

Siliceous Polishing Powder

	Parts
Zinc oxide	35
Kieselguhr	60
Pink lake	5

Mucilages convert the powders into nail-polishing pastes.

Polishing Paste

	Parts
Nail polishing powder	50
Gum tragacanth mucilage	50

By adding a mixture of wax and paraffin to the pastes they can be moulded into small sticks.

Nail-preserving Creams

Creams for the care of the nails are usually based on anhydrous or emulsified cholesterinated petroleum oils.

Cream (after F. Chilson)

	Parts
Petroleum jelly	25
Petroleum oil	25
Talcum	20
Titanium oxide	20
Zinc peroxide	7·5

Such fatty creams can so impregnate the nail that neither nail polish nor varnish will adhere to the surface. It is accordingly better to use the glycerinated creams referred to in the chapters on "Creams."

Cuticle Removers

Cuticle Remover

	Parts
Glycerine	20
Trisodium phosphate	5
Water	75
Perfume	*q.s.*
Colour	*q.s.*

Caustic alkalis are no longer used.

Acid Nail Solution

	Parts
Oxalic acid	0·25
Citric acid	9·75
Rose water	90

Acid Nail Solution (Reece Bundock)

	Parts
Oxalic acid	15
Phenylacetic acid	1
Water	1,000

Hydrogen Peroxide for Nails

	Parts
Hydrogen peroxide, 20 vols.	50
Glycerine	10
Rose water	20

Alkaline Cuticle Cream (after F. Chilson)

	Parts
Cholesterinated petroleum jelly (semi-liquid)	42
Wax	10
Sodium lauryl sulphonate	4
Trisodium phosphate	2
Water	18

A borated cold cream may also be used in conjunction with tri-sodium phosphate as the alkali.

Hand Milk

(U.S. Patent 2,436,818, November, 1948).

	Parts
Glycerine	50
Lanolin	7·5
Glycol stearate	60
Sorbitol syrup	30
Alcohol	50
Barley flour fraction	5
Water	75·25
Antiseptic	*q.s.*
Perfume	*q.s.*

INDEX